RADICAL INDULGENCE

RADICAL INDULGENCE
The Health Secrets of Coffee, Chocolate & Wine

Mary Boone Wellington

Rose Cottage Press
A Small Publishing House
in the
Great North Woods of New Hampshire

I only regret my economies...

· ·

Lady Coghill to her son Nevill on her deathbed

Contents

Studies, Science and 'Truthiness'

. . . .

Earnest scientists set out to study a myriad of substances, effects, and practices, and I believe there is a good-faith effort on the part of the initiator to get to the bottom of something and to prove or disprove a theory. Things can get confusing when the funding company or organization has a clear stake in the outcome of research to "prove" their product, service, method, or thesis is the best. For this reason, I looked carefully at each original study, the credentials of the researcher, and who provided the funding, while researching this book. Even careful diligence comes to nothing when the facts and figures are fudged, as is sometimes the case.

That said, I believe the scientific community has a bigger stake in honest and objective examination and clear conclusions than in pleasing one client or funder. There are many participants on the research side of these years-long investigations, and if there is funny business afoot, well, someone usually rats them out.

The study is one thing and the conclusions are another. Take the excitement over resveratrol. I heard about this cool substance on the news one night—some TV network guru doc was extolling the amazing properties of this breakthrough discovery. A quick Google search in the weeks that followed showed any number of places where I could get myself a supply of resveratrol. Being a bit skeptical, I read carefully and found that the suppliers' claims to have been endorsed by Oprah or Dr. Oz were almost certainly spurious. I could find no verification of dosage, resveratrol content, or any way to be certain that taking this drug would turn me into the human equivalent of a super sleek little mouse living an active and healthy life right up to the end of my days running the maze.

I refrained from ordering and delved deeper. Turns out that the interpretation of the original resveratrol study was wildly optimistic and had conveniently left out a few key facts. The dosage of resveratrol given the fat little mice in the study was 2,000 times what one would get from a glass or two of wine. The resveratrol mice in the study were indeed quite healthy active, sleek, and lovely until the day they died, fat and happy. This is a great outcome, I think, and I would love that for myself, but the claims of longevity were exaggerated. In fact, the resveratrol mice had exactly the same lifespans as their old, somewhat ragged and fat, sluggish friends.

Good-faith efforts on the part of science should be applauded, media hype and confusion aside. I am convinced there is plenty of peer scrutiny given to any research claim. In fact, I uncovered many fierce debates over what looked to me like minuscule and only moderately interesting facts. These debates sparked further inquiries and research, and while every 't' has not been crossed nor every 'i' dotted, there is plenty of good coming out of the struggle to be first on the scene with a valuable bit of science. We all benefit enormously from the efforts of the bioscience community, whether for profit or academic advancement.

The scientific community was justified in its excitement about resveratrol, for another layer of the veils between humans knowing absolutely everything about health and lifespan was advanced smartly with this research, but it was far from a miracle for those of us on the brink of what I like to call "late middle age" right now.

I understand the need to make new data into a compelling story. Getting the hopes and fears of the population all stirred up is a journalistic tradition, but sending us all out for another bottle of Ripple in the false hope it will keep us young is just a tad tragic.

In the health benefit sections that follow, I have taken into account the limitations of the trials and studies as I see them. I don't have a degree in science, but I do have a keen eye for what Stephen Colbert calls "truthiness." We want to believe, we really do, and tend to meet the charlatans halfway as they pitch their snake-oil remedies. I promise to lay out the facts without embellishment and to be as clear as I can about my own hopes, preferences, and dreams, so that you can draw your own conclusions.

Disclaimer

In this book I'm coming right out and proclaiming the virtues of coffee, chocolate, and wine, despite having been raised Methodist, where all the bottles of hooch were kept under the kitchen sink with the Clorox as though they were poison. True, there are people who should go nowhere near those three goodies for very sensible reasons. I know that alcoholism is a destroyer of lives and families; that obesity is a huge (pardon the pun) problem in the US; and that coffee, while not exactly the devil, is nevertheless banned by the Mormon Church and will keep you up past your bedtime.

I'm not saying you should eat and drink with abandon, no matter what. I'm just saying that there is a case for health benefits of coffee, chocolate, and wine as evidenced by recent research. Read, become informed, don't do anything that worries you, and above all, don't go sayin' you did it because I said it was all right. This book reflects my personal experience, position, and opinion. It is not meant to be a directive. Consider yourself warned. You are a grownup, check with your health care provider if you have doubts, and then do as you think best.

INTRODUCTION

Living It Up Without Giving It Up

. . . .

At a retreat with creative business leaders from all over the
world in a lovely decadent old hotel on the Riviera where the
rooms were luxurious, the food enticing, the wines superb and
abundant, my stand on denial began to shift. The organizer of
the retreat was a beautiful woman from the fairytale kingdom of
Monaco. As she sensuously spooned chocolate mousse through
coral lips and sipped a dark espresso, she scolded us Americans
for passing up such fine indulgences.

"In Europe, we are all very passionate about our pleasures,
almost as passionate and proud as Americans are about their
restraint." This stuck with me all these years and I have to say,
it seems more than a bit true.

I was a skeptic on the health benefits of indulgence, but
having heard the news reports of the healthy properties of some
of my favorites, I was ready for a closer look. Wondering if
the new research had been funded by the coffee, chocolate,
and wine industries, or if they were independent projects, I
gathered reports, studies, and dense scientific papers from all
over the world and dove into this tall stack of scientific reports

1

with hope in my heart, but determined to rein in my enthusiasm and make an honest assessment.

Do coffee, chocolate, and wine offer rejuvenation of body and spirit or have we been fooling ourselves, based on dubious and scant evidence? I wrote this book to share what I learned about the science behind some of our favorite indulgences and to find out once and for all the truth about them.

I went deep into the topic to find out if my delightful new vision of a life well lived with indulgence on all sides, was a fool's paradise, destined to toss me up, sad, sick, and old one day in the distant future. Or was it truly as it seemed—a sustainable way of life that fostered health and longevity?

Confused, I set out to sort through it all for myself, and thus began my burning desire to share the facts, just the facts, ma'am. Like Officer Gannon on the old Dragnet show, as much as I wanted to find the guilty party, I needed all the facts before I could draw any meaningful conclusion. As you might have guessed, I have proved to my personal satisfaction that the consumption of wine, chocolate, and coffee—*moderate* consumption—is of positive benefit to health. Moreover, it can serve, as a spiritual, mental, and emotional boost to a life that seems all too short—'way too short, now that I know I can indulge to my heart's (and I mean that quite literally) content.

At the risk of spoiling it all for you, I must reveal at the outset that the news is good, very good indeed. A life threaded with regular (and well-regulated) doses of coffee, chocolate, and wine will serve you well. No, one may not totally overdo it and remain healthy; all the good may be undone by failing to observe just a little restraint, but we can all begin to celebrate and start a new form of renunciation. We must now give up our austerities.

"Live fast, die young, and leave a beautiful corpse"

This motto, first spoken by John Derek in the movie *"Knock on any Door"* is one that served modern generations in their youth, but now may need alterating. With the prospect of out-living our forbears due to better nutrition, advanced science and our focus on feeling fit–that boat sailed long ago. I propose a new motto for Boomers:

"Play hard, indulge intelligently and don't die 'till you are good and old–then you'll die happy"

If you embrace my new motto, you will enjoy all your years, stay sharp and vigorous till the end, and possibly still leave a beautiful corpse. One thing is for certain, there will be a beatific smile on your lips as you bid farewell.

My journey from restraint to revelation began when I started to write about how to secure a happy and healthy old age, in my first book, *Hope I Don't Die Before I Get Old* with co-author Tracey Bowman. I found remarkable new research showing that desirable food and drink I never dreamed could be good for me had very real health-building qualities.

This sounded too good to be true, but reports that red wine, coffee, and chocolate were the holy trinity of youth and vigor were appearing regularly in the news. Were these cleverly disguised advertisements or gospel truth?

Having become very fit a decade before, in my early fifties, I couldn't help but notice that I had slipped. Nothing on my body was quite where I remembered it being and surely there was more of it than there should be. Returning to the same routines that delivered the miracle of my transformation from a sad, dyspeptic, vegetarian couch potato into a slim, chirpy, cheerful runner who ate salad and burgers (minus the bun—never the bun, I made a second try at renewing body and thus, soul.

The first time around, it took a mere three months of downing vitamins six times a day, running forty minutes in all weather, choking down chalky protein drinks, and resisting the cravings for just about every food except meat and green vegetables, to transform me into a woman with energy to burn and a slim, strong figure. Dropping thirty-five pounds to a size four in the process gave me the opportunity to indulge in a new wardrobe and I felt like the cat that ate the canary. Actually, canary was not mentioned as a preferred food for me, but would probably have fit well into my steady diet of turkey, beef, and wild game, with a side of greens.

When I gave this same regimen a second try a decade later, sadly, shockingly, even though I was religious about following the same instructions, I did not achieve the same results the second time around. I had not descended to my previous low, (or high, weight-wise) but I knew what it felt like to bound up stairs, then agree happily to another two-mile hike with the grandkids after my morning five-mile run. I wanted that edge I'd felt with reserves of energy to draw upon for work or fun.

I just could not get on board with the "age slows you down" concept so many of my contemporaries voiced After all, slippage notwithstanding, I felt better now at sixty-two than I had for most of my forties, so I was not about to let this insidious blah become my norm.

When the scale refused to budge, week after week and the tape measure showed no difference and my clothes continued to hitch up on my hips, I got mad. "Son of a Biscuit Eater! (or words to that effect)," I exclaimed each week at the ritual weigh-in when I saw no change in the scale. (Please note that I had not actually eaten a biscuit in years.) Stepping up my weekly curse fest at the device as I stepped on the scale proved an ineffective exercise for reducing my girth.

I began to measure with vigor, acquiring new gadgets to monitor my efforts. Abandoning my rigorous routine for those even more restrictive, I even tried Weight Watchers for two weeks. I morphed into the Weight Watcher Nazi, measuring and weighing all my portions and being super vigilant about all my records. Calculators were employed. Charts were made. Special foods with the point value printed on them were purchased. Austerities were observed.

And then—a major hissy fit on discovering that, after two weeks of this rigor, I had actually gained two pounds. I know, I know, most people have great results with the program; I must have a hormone or thyroid problem, I thought. So I went and got tested and—no such luck. It was a bit cheering to find out exactly how healthy I was: everything in balance, bad cholesterol low, good cholesterol high, thyroid OK, no hormonal issues, heart strong, no suspicious spots—and no excuses. Drat!

What does all this have to do with coffee, chocolate, and wine? Why am I telling you all about my abstinence? Because I proved to myself that abstinence was not necessary to achieve the goals I cherished! Austerity and abstinence brought nothing more than a tight inner Puritan smile. While my ancestors did not come over on the Mayflower seeking satisfaction in a life of limited resources, my family has been here for twelve generations, and the Puritan "all work and no pleasure" ethic has had its effect. I have the dearly held belief that if I like it, crave it, enjoy it in any way, then it is definitely BAD for me.

With all the focus on healthy lifestyles, the Mediterranean diet seems to be most often recommended as the best for health and longevity. After all my attempts to shock my body back into its slim (possibly too slim) former glory, I swapped the scale and austerity for a focus on building health and strength by eating in a healthy and satisfying way. (After all, I had given restraint my best shot, with depressing results.) This includes a cup or two of my favorite espresso in the morning, an ounce or two of dark chocolate as the fancy strikes me, and a glass of dark red wine every evening. With these treats coming my way regularly, isn't too hard to stick to a healthy eating plan on a daily basis.

I find that by spending one day cooking up a week's supply of delicious, healthful, good-for-me foods, I stick to those foods all week. One giant vegetable frittata gives me a fast and complete breakfast each morning, no matter how rushed I am. A pot of spiced vegetables with generous lashings of olive oil and a roasted beast of some kind forms the basis of lunch or dinner when I am too busy to notice mealtime is upon me. Without my healthy supply in the fridge, I would be snacking on less satisfying fare, ingesting twice the calories and half the nutrition along the way.

There is a time and a place for everything, so every weekend I make bread and eat all I want. I have learned how to bake brioche, my favorite, and crusty baguettes, yum! What is better than a feast of bread warm from the oven, slathered in butter and eaten without guilt? One day a week, I give myself permission to eat absolutely anything I want, however decadent. Guess what? The novelty wears off. Now I find myself eating only one or two crazy foods, like pizza with cake on "feast day."

Currently a big plate of French fries cooked in duck fat is my favorite treat. Sometimes I have waffles for dinner with maple syrup, pecans, whipped cream and all. Then I go right back to my healthy staples for the rest of the week. I have proven to myself what slim, strong European women have known all along. If you eat a diet that satisfies your nutritional needs while including sensuous details in a way that maximizes their enjoyment, then you will be a happy camper, not needing to eat a whole bag of cookies in the dark to fill up the loose and ragged ends of desire.

How is my new regimen working out for me? In spite of a winter spent writing all day and experimenting with new truffle recipes for my next book (a cookbook for healthy treats featuring,–you guessed it–coffee, chocolate, and wine as star ingredients), I am back in shape. Not as slim as I was at my low ten years before, but, as I mentioned, perhaps I was too slim then. I am strong, feel energetic, and am entering what I like to call "late middle age" with all the style, vigor, and enthusiasm I need.

Just last week I bought a new backpack and boots, camp stove, and sleeping bag and began to download trail maps for my second leg of the Pacific Crest trail trek next summer. Forty years ago I hiked the Oregon section of the PCT—all 430 miles, from the southern border of Washington to California's northern one. It was the worst and best experience of my young life up till then (I was only twenty-three.)

Since then I have married, had three children, divorced, launched four companies, flirted with chronic fatigue syndrome, and lived to tell the tale.

I'm ready to hit the trail again next summer. I may have to step up the pace if I'm to complete the 2,663-mile length of the Pacific Crest Trail by the time I fall off the perch. If anyone out there knows how to freeze dry wine, please let me know, for the toughest conceptual challenge as I plan is the thought of having to forgo my daily glass or two.

So, read this book and arm yourself with the facts. Then, Readers, go forth and INDULGE! Spread the word to your poor chocolate, coffee, and wine-starved friends, and you will have a much happier group of companions with whom to grow old.

The problem with people who have no vices is that generally you can be pretty sure they're going to have some pretty annoying virtues.

....

Elizabeth Taylor

Coffee

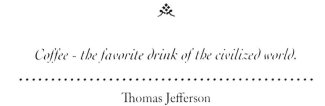

Coffee - the favorite drink of the civilized world.

Thomas Jefferson

Chapter 1

First Things First

· ·

Coffee was a staple in my home growing up. An enduring memory of the little house on School Street was the smell and sound of coffee percolating at quarter past four every morning as my grandparents prepared to go to work. Both my grandparents had government jobs and got an early jump on their commute. Starting their shifts at 6:00 a.m. meant they could beat the traffic—fierce even back then—and be home before the afternoon rush hour. The coffee must have helped with this early-bird special, but they drank coffee all day long, just for the pleasure of it. If my grandfather couldn't sleep, he often got up, made himself a cup of instant, and went back to bed. What a constitution!

I got to sample the stuff on road trips where a scalding brew was poured from a Scotch thermos, thinned with lots of milk and sugar and given to me as a treat by the side of the road. It was not bad, but seemed a dangerous substance, so hot even with the milk that it required tiny sips and much blowing across the top. I marveled at how my grandmother could drink her scalding hot cup right down. Once the snack was done, thermos recorked, and the box of Uneeda Biscuits stowed, we were on our way again, headed for "the country," as we called the home place in the Tidewater region of Virginia.

This was a special treat for the road. Children in our family rarely got a sip of coffee, as it was not considered good for growing bodies. It was not until I was a teenager studying art that I started to drink coffee in earnest. It began one evening at a new class I had signed up for at my summer art school. People of all ages attended this local institution, run by a Washington Color School painter, Ed McGowan. Local artists of some renown were teachers there—my first introduction to the economic necessities of a glamorous career in the arts.

I had signed up for a class called "Life Drawing" and thought I was in for some instruction on drawing pears, vases, maybe a dead fowl or flower. People were milling around, setting up their big pads of paper and getting out their charcoal, when a lovely little woman of a certain age—as the French say about people they view as no longer young but not yet "old,"—arrived from the back room and took her place on the raised platform in the center. She was wearing a kimono and I thought, cool, we get to draw people. Just about that time, she dropped her robe and sat on the stool, bare naked for all to see.

I'm pretty sure I dropped my charcoal and headed for the back of the room where I busied myself with the coffee pot. Not being a coffee drinker, I decided on the spot I would take it black—it seemed more sophisticated and grown up. It was a decision I soon regretted, for it left me nothing to do but return to my easel with my steaming, bitter brew in hand and attempt to peep around the edge of my drawing pad at the spectacle before me.

The teacher must have noticed my failure to observe, pick up my charcoal, or make a mark, and he eventually got around to suggesting I try to draw an "ant's journey" all around the edge of the body before me. I did, but the progress was slow and hesitant. I drank cup after cup of the truly horrible coffee to kill time and waited out the two hours of the class—two hours! By 9:00 p.m. I was having a sort of out-of-body experience from all the caffeine, but felt I had covered my lack of worldliness pretty well. Sure, I was awake till 4:00 a.m.– felt simultaneously wired and exhausted the next day, but I was exhilarated by the double achievement of having survived my first life drawing class and my first bout of coffee consumption. I was ready for more of both.

Chapter 2

Where It All Began

. . . .

The first coffee was brewed in Ethiopia in the 11th century. Considered medicinal, only the leaves were boiled for a brew offering doubtful pleasures. There is a lot of lore about the plants being discovered by a Turkish goatherd who noticed how lively his flock became after eating the red coffee "cherries." Eventually, folks caught onto fermenting the fruit, removing the bean or seed, and roasting it for a brew similar to what we know as coffee. Before long, shops seling coffee sprang up all over Turkey and coffeehouses became cultural meeting places where the intelligentsia went to discuss business and culture, to read and exchange ideas.

Coffee became the popular beverage for royalty and soon a royal coffee brewer post was established in the Ottoman Empire. Brought to Venice in the 1600s by merchants who had enjoyed it in Istanbul, coffee took off in Italy. It then became suspect and was denounced as the drink of the Devil–until the Pope got a taste and proclaimed it "good." Thus coffee was launched in the west. The first European coffee house—Café de Procope—was established and soon there was one on every corner in Paris.

Before long, coffee was sparking conversation and trade, all over Europe and finally in Vienna. Having defeated and chased off the Turks, the Viennese found among their abandoned supplies 500 sacks of coffee (clearly an army that had its priorities straight, if not its fighting prowess) and concluded that the stuff was camel fodder. Luckily, a gentleman who had spent time in Turkey heard of the bounty; he soon acquired the sacks and taught the Viennese to brew and enjoy coffee. They didn't have many camels anyway, so, just as well.

From there, coffee spread to every corner of the world, and enterprising pioneers begged, borrowed, and stole seeds and plants to cultivate all over equatorial regions of the new world. Following the Boston tea party, coffee emerged as the top beverage in the Americas, as it is today. Worldwide, tea is still the most widely drunk beverage, but coffee is gaining, even in China.

The joke was, President Bush only declared war when Starbucks was hit. You can mess with the U.N. all you want, but when you start interfering with the right to get caffeinated, someone has to pay.

Chris Kyle

RADICAL INDULGENCE

Chapter 3

How Coffee Is Grown

. . . .

Coffee is grown in over fifty countries, mostly around the equator. It is grown on low bushes in the shade of rainforest trees, the preferred environment. There, among a variety of plants, ally insects and plants repel the enemies of the coffee plant. On a sustainable coffee farm, the beans (which are really a fruit) are harvested when ripe, soaked and hulled, then sorted for size. The biggest beans are considered the finest, and they are bagged green for export to the coffee roastary. Saved to use as compost on around the coffee trees, the hulls serve as both fertilizer and weed killer.

When coffee growers want to produce a bigger crop, they plant coffee trees all together in a monoculture with no forest friends or shade. That means pesticides and fertilizers must be used to ensure a crop of beans. Up to 3,000 pounds of coffee can be yielded per square acre of plantation on these factory coffee farms. By contrast, coffee grown the sustainable traditional way yields only 450 to 900 pounds per acre. Sounds sensible to clear and plant, but there is a high price to pay for such productivity.

After tobacco and cotton, conventionally produced coffee is the third most heavily chemically treated crop in the world. Some of the synthetic pesticides and fertilizers used on the cultivated coffee crops are banned in most western nations, and they're often used without any genuine regulatory supervision.

There is debate on how many of the chemicals used on nonorganic coffee make their way into the bean and survive the roasting process, but there is one way to be certain you are not ingesting these chemicals: buy only organic coffee.

In addition to the impact on your body, the process of growing coffee in a nonorganic way is killing off vast populations of songbirds. The songbirds, which have a huge migratory territory, have been decreasing in number since the 1940s.

If your concern for the birds is not stirring you to action on the organic coffee front, consider the plight of the coffee plantation worker, whose exposure to the toxic chemicals can be fatal, especially to children, who often work alongside their parents.

Consider looking for "fair trade coffee." When we fork over what seems like shocking amounts of money for our fancy coffee, only about ten percent of that cash makes its way back to the farmers who do all the work. By buying fair trade coffee, you are helping to build the market for a fine product, grown with earth-friendly, sustainable techniques, and supporting a fair wage for those who labor for your pleasure. The fair trade premium supports the communities where the farms are located and ensures a living wage to the workers there, along with hope for the future.

Coffee must be picked at just the right moment. Remember that Juan Valdez commercial? Juan was carefully fingering a small cluster of coffee cherries, as the fruit is called. One must wait till the fruit is perfectly ripe for the finest coffee, and that does not happen all at once. To harvest each future bean at its peak is a risky business and more of an art and labor of love than just firing up the combine and rolling down a row of plants.

One such coffee company is the Conti Gourmet Coffee Company. A family business for three generations, this coffee producer practices sustainable farming with it's shady planta-tions and organic methods. They do this to preserve the quality of their product and to ensure the company thrives for the next generation. I love the idea of supporting such an artisan venture halfway around the world.

If none of these socially conscious ideals move you, think about this. In supporting traditional methods of coffee culti-vation by buying organic fair trade brews, you are ensuring a supply of delicious, unique flavors for your coffee drinking years. Let the gourmand inside you loose and pony up the extra dough in the name of self-interest.

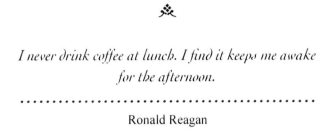

I never drink coffee at lunch. I find it keeps me awake for the afternoon.

Ronald Reagan

Chapter 4

Good for What Ails You

. . . .

Coffee has been getting a bad rap for a long time. Seems that some of the early studies showing a negative effect failed to adjust for a few little details, such as smoking, While they showed a definite correlation between coffee drinking and increased risk for heart disease, they failed to note that the riskiest drinkers in their study were also smoking, along with their coffee.

Once the studies narrowed their focus, coffee began its long road to a complete image makeover from culprit to hero. Now we hear all about how good coffee is for you, but the shadow of the old reports and recommendations still lingers.

Approached at a conference by a very earnest holistic physician who worried that my new book might lure unsuspecting future heart-attack victims down a delicious and stimulating road to ruin, I assured him I was doing my homework. When I asked my assistants to bring me some data on the health benefits of coffee, it took four tries to get them pointed at the positive viewpoint, so prevalent was the idea that it must be bad. I reviewed the negative findings and found them to be flawed and outdated in most cases.

Consider your overall health picture. If you have chronic health problems, please note that the tests and studies showing both the benefits and harm of coffee were done on healthy folks, people who do not confront the challenges you may face. And here is one very real note of caution: the way your coffee is prepared can affect your health. If high cholesterol or too much LDL cholesterol is a problem for you, then drink only filtered coffee. For some reason, unfiltered coffee can raise cholesterol levels.

A 2010 study found that regular coffee consumption increased total cholesterol, but much of this rise in blood lipids was due to an increase in the "good" cholesterol, HDL. The LDL ("bad" cholesterol) to HDL ratio actually improved. This suggests that coffee intake may offer cardiovascular protection in those with low to normal total cholesterol and low HDL. Cafestol and kahweol, the coffee compounds believed to cause these effects, are highest in unfiltered coffee.

As with all your indulgences, watch out for collateral damage. Drinking your four cups a day with cream, sugar, flavored syrup, and whipped cream might tip the balance of healthy beverage to dangerous treat!

 Let me be clear. Coffee is not for everyone and not everyone should drink four cups a day for health. If, however, after reviewing the facts, coffee turns out to be more of a help than a harm to you, I will be pleased to have brought the good news your way.

Tea has many of the healthy qualities of coffee and may be a good choice for you if your body does not tolerate coffee. Michael Harney of Harney Tea Company has written a terrific book on the topic-*The Harney & Sons Guide to Tea.* Stop in to their SoHo, NY shop for a cup of tea and a copy and pick up a stylish tin of your favorite brew while you are there. I love the Dragon Pearl Jasmine and their Irish Breakfast is perfection.

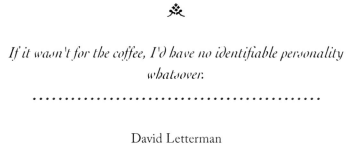

If it wasn't for the coffee, I'd have no identifiable personality whatsover.

. . . .

David Letterman

Chapter 5

Coffee and Heart Disease

· ·

In a meta study— one in which past research is reviewed and then included or excluded to garner new conclusions from the combined efforts of many researchers and studies—researchers Elizabeth Mostofsky, Megan S. Rice, Emily B. Levitan, and Murray A. Mittleman concluded that "Moderate coffee consumption is inversely associated with risk of heart failure, with the largest inverse association observed for consumption of four servings per day." Reported in 2012 in the publication *Circulation: Heart Failure*, (published by the American Heart Association), the study assessed the relationship between habitual coffee consumption and the risk of heart failure.

The researchers made a meticulous compilation of data on 6,522 heart failure events among 140,220 participants. In the end, they recommended modifying the earlier recommendation that coffee is harmful to the heart by saying, "Coffee may, in fact, may provide moderate protection against heart failure incidence."

Chapter 6

Coffee and Cancer

. . . .

There was a time, not too long ago, when just about everything you tried to ingest was suspected of causing cancer. It's nice to hear some good news for a change about a substance we have relied on for centuries for energy, comfort, and joy.

A few good reasons to drink coffee are reduced risk of brain, uterine, prostate, head and oral, colon, liver, and breast cancer. That is a pretty big claim. I looked into these reports, sometimes relayed by coffee-promoting "news" agencies, and investigated them for authenticity, and guess what? They all checked out as real science.

Sure, there was a certain amount of exaggeration, but for the most part, they are accurate claims. Should you step up your coffee intake to prevent cancer? That's up to you, but at the very least, you can feel good about your habit for some very sound scientific reasons. "There are estimated to be over a couple thousand different components in coffee, many of which are antioxidants," says Donald Hensrud, MD, Chair of Preventive Medicine at the Mayo Clinic in Rochester, Minnesota.

Here is the scoop on coffee and cancer by type. I'm listing only the research that showed conclusive results here.

Brain Cancer
Researchers in the UK examined the coffee-drinking habits of 300 cancer patients and compared them to 300 cancer-free people. They found that among those who drank at

least five cups of caffeinated coffee per day, there was less chance of developing gliomas, a type of brain cancer. They postulate that the caffeine, which restricts blood flow to the brain, caused the cancer cells to be deprived of the oxygen and nutrients they needed to survive. I'm no scientist, but what does logic say about the normal brain cells getting the oxygen and nutrients they need to survive as well? Something to think about.

Uterine Cancer

Researchers found, in a study at Harvard University of 67, 470 women between the ages of thirty-four and fifty-nine, that women who routinely drank several cups of coffee per day had a 25 percent lower risk of developing uterine cancer than those who did not drink coffee. The study spanned twenty-six years.

Coffee is a rich source of antioxidants, including polyphenols, even more than are found in tea, and it seems that with coffee, the more, the better. Studies found that women drinking four or more cups a day had a 25 percent lower risk of developing endometrial cancer than women who did not drink coffee. Women drinking two to three cups per day had a 14 percent lower risk.

While researchers fall short of recommending that women take up the coffee habit, they note that there are few side effects to drinking four cups of coffee per day, save insomnia and possibly heartburn. Choose low-acid types of coffee to reduce the heartburn. Brazilian coffee is generally the lowest acid coffee, with Sumatran next in acid content. One brand, PuRoast, has less than half the acid found in Starbucks coffee.

Prostate Cancer

Coffee contains many biologically active compounds, such as antioxidants and minerals. Current research has not isolated the contributing factors, but it seems there is a link between coffee consumption and lowered risk of prostate cancer, including lethal and advanced types.

Kathryn M. Wilson, PhD, a postdoctoral fellow at the Channing Laboratory, Harvard Medical School, and the Harvard School of Public Health, reports that "Coffee has effects on insulin and glucose metabolism as well as sex hormone levels, all of which play a role in prostate cancer. It was plausible that there may be an association between coffee and prostate cancer."

Cancer risk was lowered by 60 percent among men who drank the most coffee. Researchers determined that caffeine is not a key factor in the cancer prevention effect, so decaf is a good choice for those concerned with sleeplessness.

Oral and Head Cancer

By pooling an analysis of nine different studies, researchers at the International Head and Neck Cancer Epidemiology (IN-HANCE) consortium found good outcomes for regular coffee drinkers. By drinking four or more cups of coffee per day, participants in the studies were found to have a 39 percent lower risk of oral and pharynx cancers (combined).

They did not have enough data on decaffeinated coffee but believe that decaffeination is not a detriment to the anticancer effect. Lead researcher Mia Hashibe, PhD, assistant professor in the department of family and preventive medicine at the University of Utah, Salt Lake City, and a Huntsman Cancer

Institute investigator, tells us, "Since coffee is so widely used and there is a relatively high incidence and low survival rate of these forms of cancers, our results have important public health implications that need to be further addressed. What makes our results so unique is that we had a very large sample size, and since we combined data across many studies, we had more statistical power to detect associations between cancer and coffee."

Colon Cancer

Dr. Rashmi Sinha, the lead author of a National Cancer Institute study of more than half a million Americans, looked at dietary habits and health and found that people who drank over four cups of coffee per day—both regular and decaf—had a 15 percent lower risk of developing colon cancer. Although the fifteen-plus-year study was thorough, adjusting subjects' profiles for weight, exercise, history of cancer, and alcohol use, researchers were unable to find the specific cause for this effect.

A component in coffee called methylpyridinium that offers protection from colon cancer, was isolated and identified by at the Institute for Food Chemistry at the University of Munster in Germany in 2003. This substance is found almost exclusively in coffee and coffee products, but is not found in significant amounts in other foods and beverages.

Study leaders Thomas Hofmann, PhD, professor and head of the Institute for Food Chemistry at the University of Munster in Germany, and Veronika Somoza, PhD, deputy director of the German Research Center for Food Chemistry in Garching, say that "Until human studies are done, no one knows exactly how much coffee is needed to have a protective effect against colon cancer," adding, "however, our studies suggest that drinking coffee may offer some protection, especially if it's strong. For example, espresso-type coffee contains about two to three times more of the anticancer compound than a medium-roasted coffee beverage."

Colon cancer is one of the easiest cancers to cure if caught early enough. Get screened for colon cancer at forty if you have a family history, and fifty if not, then every ten years after that.

Liver Cancer

Cancer of the liver is the third greatest cause of death from cancer worldwide. Researchers examining studies in southern European countries, where coffee is enjoyed extensively, and also in countries where it is less common, like Japan, have concluded that there is a lower risk among coffee drinkers for liver cancer. Compared to noncoffee drinkers, those who enjoyed the beverage had a 41 percent lower risk of liver cancer.

How to cut your cancer risk in half? In a study of more than 90,000 Japanese by the Monami Inoue of the National Cancer Center in Tokyo, researchers looked at a ten-year study to see if coffee use was a factor in being diagnosed with liver cancer. They determined that the test subjects who drank coffee daily had half the cancer risk of those who never drank coffee.

Breast Cancer

The role of coffee in delaying the onset of, or eliminating the risk of breast cancer has been researched by the Lund University and Malmö University in Sweden. Coffee is known to affect the metabolization of estrogen in women with certain types of genes called CYP1A2. Women who had one of the C-type genes and drank three cups of coffee per day developed breast cancer much less frequently than women with the same gene who did not drink coffee. Their risk of cancer was only two-thirds that of the noncoffee-drinking women. These research findings are published in the journal *Cancer Epidemiology*, Biomarkers and Prevention, with doctoral student Erika Bågeman as lead author.

About 25 percent of all breast cancers are estrogen-receptor negative (ER-negative).. Swedish researchers at the Karolinska Institutet, found that by drinking five cups of coffee per day, risk factors were lowered by 57 percent. Even after taking into account family history, diet, body mass, and hormone replacement therapy, this held true. The study involved 6,000 Swedish women and although it does not point to the causes for the results, I think they are impressive enough to up my coffee intake.

Tumor Growth and Coffee

Coffee is also known to slow the growth of tumors, another factor in its effectiveness against cancer. New research published in the 2011 journal *Breast Cancer Research*, says that the effects of coffee consumption may inhibit certain types of fast growing and more lethal breast cancers.

It should be noted that the caffeine in coffee can cause painful effects for women suffering benign breast cysts and that in this case, giving up coffee will often relieve the symptoms.

※

I make a mean cup of coffee, if you give me the right ingredients.

....

Ice Cube

Chapter 7

Coffee and Diabetes

. . . .

Type 2 diabetes afflicts 10.9 million Americans, which is 26.9 percent of the US population, according to the US Department of Health and Human Services in 2011. Anything that can be done to protect against this deadly disease should receive serious attention. Coffee has been the subject of extensive scrutiny as a preventative for type 2 diabetes, the most common form of diabetes.

In type 2 diabetes, either the body does not produce enough insulin or the cells ignore the insulin. Naturally produced by the healthy body, insulin is used to break down sugars, and when this is lacking, the glucose (sugar) builds up in cells, causing diabetic complications such as glaucoma, cataracts, neuropathy and skin infections.

High-glucose tolerance has been observed in habitual coffee users. Research using data from several studies was done by the Department of Nutrition, Harvard School of Public Health, Boston, Massachusetts. They looked at the correlation between coffee use and prevention of diabetes.

The test subjects were 86,259 women, ages twenty-six to forty-six, with no history of diabetes. The variables were adjusted to take into account body weight, variations in quantity, types of coffee (decaf and instant included), and other lifestyle risks, such as smoking and alcohol consumption. The study concluded that there was a reduction of risk in the group that consumed coffee on a regular basis over a ten-year follow-up, and that the risk was substantially lower among the younger members of the study.

Looking into the causes for this reduced risk, researchers at UCLA discovered the molecular mechanism that might possibly be behind coffee's protective effect.

A protein called sex hormone-binding globulin (SHBG) regulates the biological activity of the body's sex hormones—testosterone and estrogen—which have long been thought to play a role in the development of type 2 diabetes. Coffee consumption, it turns out, increases plasma levels of SHBG.

Atsushi Goto, a UCLA doctoral student in epidemiology, and Dr. Simin Liu, a professor of epidemiology and medicine with joint appointments at the UCLA School of Public Health and the David Geffen School of Medicine at UCLA, have demonstrated in their new research that women who drink at least four cups of coffee a day are less than half as likely to develop diabetes as noncoffee drinkers.

The researchers have also identified two mutations on the gene for SHBG that indicate a risk for diabetes. "It seems that SHBG in the blood does reflect a genetic susceptibility to developing type 2 diabetes" Liu said. "but we now further show that this protein can be influenced by dietary factors."

One bit of possible bad news is that they found no change in the SHBG levels in decaf drinkers. "Consumption of decaffeinated coffee was not significantly associated with SHBG levels, nor diabetes risk," Goto said. "So you probably have to go for the octane!"

Wait, I'm going out for another cup of coffee—this is pretty compelling stuff; I want to be sharp enough to take it all in!

It is inhumane, in my opinion, to force people who have a genuine medical need for coffee to wait in line behind people who apparently view it as some kind of recreational activity.

. . . .

Dave Barry

Chapter 8

Coffee and Stroke

. . . .

Here is a report that came out at exactly the right time. According to a recent article published in the journal *Neurology*, drinking coffee "transiently increases the risk of ischemic stroke onset, particularly among infrequent drinkers." This was reported in the Harvard Crimson just before exams began at the University!

Students might well wonder and worry as they drink cup after cup to stay up while cramming data into their heads to achieve the high grades they need to stay at Harvard. They needn't worry for few college age students are candidates for this type of stroke as it turns out.

In the study, researchers from the Harvard School of Public Health, Harvard Medical School, and the University of North Carolina School of Public Health examined the coffee-drinking habits of stroke survivors. Subjects were asked whether they drank coffee during the last year and if they had consumed coffee in the hour before stroke onset. As it turns out, that last cup of coffee consumed in the hour before the stroke's onset doubled the risk of stroke in the test subjects. Unlucky timing, I'd say.

On the other hand, the American Heart Association magazine *Stroke* reported that in a Swedish study of 34, 670 women without a history of cardiovascular disease or cancer, low or no coffee consumption is associated with an increased risk of stroke in women.

In another study published in *Stroke* of about 83,000 subjects suggests that drinking green tea or coffee daily might lower stroke risk by about 20 percent, with even more protection against a specific type of stroke. "Daily drinking [of] green tea and coffee is a benefit in preventing stroke," said lead researcher Dr. Yoshihiro Kokubo, chief doctor in the department of preventive cardiology at the National Cerebral and Cardiovascular Center, in Osaka. After following test subjects for thirteen years, Dr. Kokubo found that those drinking at least one cup of coffee per day lowered their risk of stroke by abut 20 percent.

Just a note about the green tea: it has far less caffeine than coffee but still gives a lift. I quaff a couple of cups of fragrant jasmine green tea first thing in the morning because I enjoy its delicate flavor. The low dose of caffeine starts me off gently untill I stir around enough to get my espresso made.

Dr. Kokubo determined that the more green tea one drinks, the lower the risk of stroke! He notes that the effect is a little different from coffee-containing compounds known as catechins, which help regulate blood pressure and help improve blood flow. The compounds also seem to promote an anti-inflammatory effect.

One type of stroke is a hemorrhagic stroke, in which a blood vessel in the brain bursts and blood floods part of the brain. The risk for this type of stroke was cut by 32 percent among those who drank a cup of coffee or two cups of green tea daily. About 13 percent of strokes are hemorrhagic strokes, the researchers noted.

A study led by Dr. David Liebeskind, associate neurology director at the UCLA Stroke Center, which was reported at the American Stroke Association's International

Stroke Conference 2009, concluded that symptoms of stroke or transient ischemic attack are "far less common" in people who drink six cups of coffee or more per day.

❊

Television is not real life. In real life people actually have to leave the coffee shop and go to jobs.

. . . .

Bill Gates

Chapter 9

Coffee and Alzheimer's

. . . .

Who hasn't worried and wondered if Alzheimer's disease loomed in their future? What would you do? How would you be cared for? In the US alone, 5.2 million people are afflicted with this disease and, as lifespans increase, so does the chance you might develop Alzheimer's. If there were a way to prevent this, everyone would surely leap at it.

Let me define a few terms, as it all gets pretty confusing, even to folks without any of the symptoms of this brain disease. Middle Age Muddle or Old Timers Disease—the normal evolution of a brain as it ages—is what people worry may be the precursor to Alzheimer's, such as when they misplace their keys or forget to feed the dog. While there are changes to the brain that come with age, not all are bad changes, and events such as those can be considered a sign you have shifted into a more "executive" type of thinking. In this mode, both sides of the brain are utilized and sometimes it can seem that you are forgetting your own name as the brain forges new pathways. The conclusions drawn from this kind of thinking are a reflection of true wisdom. Try not to worry, go with the flow.

Folks with mild cognitive impairment (MCI) show memory loss, usually short term, but can generally function and perform daily activities. People with MCI might put their keys in the freezer, their ice cream in the cupboard and feed the dog with cat food. No real harm done, except that this condition often slides into Alzheimer's disease in a few years.

People who have mild to moderate Alzheimer's disease often have difficulty with familiar tasks. They make a cup of coffee, forget to drink it and then go make another one, which they forget to drink. Sometimes they forget simple words like toothbrush. They can become lost easily, even in their own neighborhood and may dress inappropriately, putting on all the skirts in the closet at once, for example or a parka in summer. The person with Alzheimer's disease might forget how a key works and wonder where that nice doggie came from, when it is his own pooch of ten years.

Dementia is not a single disease, but a collection of disorders of the brain. Alzheimer's is a form of dementia. A new study postulates that some folks diagnosed with Alzheimer's disease actually suffer from alcoholic dementia. This is a good reason to drink with caution, especially in the later years when the effects of alcohol can be greater.

Recent studies show that slowing brain degeneration might be as simple as adding a cup or two of coffee to your daily routine to keep your mind sharp. A study of 124 older adults who already had mild cognitive impairment found a definite correlation between coffee and caffeine consumption and preventing the onset of dementia and Alzheimer's disease.

Researchers found that test subjects who did progress to Alzheimer's had lower caffeine levels than those who did not. Their findings are published in the June 5 issue of *Journal of Alzheimer's Disease*.

They concluded that drinking three cups of caffeinated coffee per day offered some protection to degeneration of the brain. Study author Dr. Chuanhai Cao, a neuroscientist at the University of South Florida's Health Byrd Alzheimer's Institute, said in a written statement. "The results from this study, along with our earlier studies in Alzheimer's mice, are very consistent in indicating that moderate daily caffeine/coffee intake throughout adulthood should appreciably protect against Alzheimer's disease later in life."

While caffeine seems to be a big component of many studies proving that coffee protects against Alzheimer's Disease, another substance called GCSF (granulocyte colony stimulating factor) is increased in the bloodstream by the presence of caffeine. The USF Health Byrd Alzheimer's Institute is investigating GCSF treatment to prevent full-blown Alzheimer's in patients with mild cognitive impairment, a condition preceding the disease.

"Caffeinated coffee provides a natural increase in blood GCSF levels," said USF neuroscientist Dr. Chuanhai Cao, lead author of the study. "The exact way that this occurs is not understood. There is a synergistic interaction between caffeine and some mystery component of coffee that provides this beneficial increase in blood GCSF levels."

The "moderate amounts" of coffee that appear to be the minimum are still high by some people's standards—four to five cups a day—but they appear necessary to protect against Alzheimer's disease. Coffee is safe to drink in that amount and is more effective than any other known treatment, such as physical and mental exercise.

"We are not saying that daily moderate coffee consumption will completely protect people from getting Alzheimer's disease," Dr. Cao said. "However, we do believe that moderate coffee consumption can appreciably reduce your risk of this dreaded disease or delay its onset."

Drug treatments for Alzheimer's are being sought by pharmaceutical companies, but there may now be something we can do ourselves to defend against degenerative mind disease— drink more coffee!

I believe humans get a lot done, not because we're smart, but because we have thumbs so we can make coffee.

....

Flash Rosenberg

Chapter 10

Coffee and Depression

. . . .

Coffee lovers around the world know it, and now science confirms that a couple of cups of coffee a day can keep depression at bay. A report published in 2011 confirms that Harvard School of Medicine researchers, studying 50,000 women, concluded that women who drank coffee regularly showed a 15 percent lower chance of suffering depression.

"A couple of past studies found similar results," says Daniel Evatt, PhD, a psychiatry research fellow at the Johns Hopkins School of Medicine in Baltimore, who was not involved in the new research. "This study validates the association, and it was done in the best possible way."

In research investigating the relationship between coffee consumption and suicide, researchers report that along with stimulating the central nervous system, caffeine acts as a mild antidepressant by boosting the production of particular neurotransmitters in the brain. These include noradrenaline, dopamine, and serotonin. They add that this could explain the results of studies in the past that have linked the consumption of coffee to a lower risk of depression.

I know the world looks better to me after a cup or two. When my morning espresso awaits me in the kitchen, I have a reason to get up, get dressed, and head on down. After my coffee, all things seem possible and I suddenly have the energy and wits to jump into my busy day.

Chapter 11

Coffee and Endurance

· ·

Will coffee give you the strength to complete the Ironman or just survive a day with your five grandsons, all under the age of five? The answer is yes! But only if you were just about able to complete the Ironman on your own or survive the afternoon with the kids anyway.

Studies show that the caffeine will increase endurance, a needed component of both the those challenges, and the time one can continue forward in an athletic endeavor. It will not increase your overall strength, just your ability to keep on trying.

Caffeine, or 1,3,7-trimethylxanthine, is the world's most consumed natural pharmacologic agent. Coffee has been consumed since the 1500s and is the world's most popular caffeine-delivery system. Before there was coffee at every Starbucks on every corner and on every kitchen counter in the land, people got their fix straight from the plant, chewing the leaves to get the boost needed to survive.

How much more pleasant for us to engage in our daily coffee ritual! It is somewhat ironic that we think of our coffee time as a relaxing break when its effect is to make us work all the harder (and longer).

As to using caffeine to extend your athletic prowess, studies have reported discrepancies in results. Over all, the best and most consistent results are from consuming caffeine tablets, rather than coffee or energy drinks containing caffeine. This is possibly due to the wide range of caffeine content in each cup. Roast times, brew method, and even evaporation have made the calculation of caffeine in each brand and size of cup hard to predict. If you are shooting for results you can count on, then go with the tablets.

Please note this word of caution. Subjects taking a double dose hoping for extra energy, found their performance, both in terms of longevity and achievement, fell back to the uncaffeinated levels. The recommended dose for increased performance is 3 to 3.5 milligrams. More will slow you down.

What about the recovery period? Every athlete knows the importance of proper hydration and nutrition in the recovery period. For people trying to build their strength, this is really where all the action takes place. Exercise puts stress on muscle and bone, actually breaking and tearing them down. In the recovery period, extra muscle fiber and bone are laid down to be ready for the next exercise period. This is why you gain in strength when you exercise. Additional blood supply in the form of more capillaries affords a continual strengthening flow to muscles during future exercise.

Adding caffeine to the carbohydrates and vitamins in the "after exertion" period aids by increasing glycogen production by about 66 percent, thus shortening the recovery period.

Creatine, a performance-enhancing component of muscle that has been proven to increase strength and muscle performance (but not endurance), seems like a perfect pairing with caffeine, which increases endurance but not performance. Oddly, some studies show that when the two are taken together, the caffeine knocks out the creatine's ability to boost performance. Other studies are unable to show these results, so we will just have to wait for more results to form an opinion.

If you are shooting for peak athletic performance, here are the points to remember:

> • Take 3 to 6 milligrams of caffeine per kilogram body weight
> • Use a pill if you really really need to count on the results
> • Begin caffeine use sixty minutes before and continue, if possible, during performance.
> • Try the dosage out before your big day in similar conditions to fine-tune your results..
> • If you are really, really dedicated, clear your body of caffeine for a week before your feat of athletic prowess to maximize the effect.

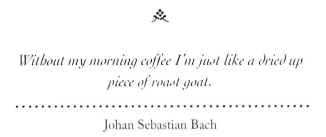

Without my morning coffee I'm just like a dried up piece of roast goat.

Johan Sebastian Bach

Chapter 12

Going Cold Turkey

· ·

Should you decide that a life with caffeine is not for you and you routinely take in more than six milligrms per day, try to taper off before going cold turkey. If you don't, the resulting head-ache can be fierce. Other side effects of quitting all at once are:

- Depression
- Fatigue
- Irritability
- Nausea and vomiting
- Muscle pain

Symptoms usually begin within eighteen hours of your last caffeine fix but are mercifully brief, peaking at twenty-four to forty-eight hours.

Pay close attention to your nutrition and hydration while quitting caffeine. Frequent high-protein meals or snacks will stabilize blood sugar and taking a multivitamin might help as well. Stay hydrated, as this helps just about every system in your body function well.

Wondering how much caffeine you are getting daily in your beverages of choice? Here is a handy guide. Remember that caffeine totals vary a good deal cup to cup, so note your sensitivity and act accordingly. The side effects of too much caffeine—jumpiness, anxiety, and racing heart—are not fun and can be dangerous.

Cola—12oz.............................. 35-55 mg
Hot brewed tea—8oz....................40-60 mg
Instant ice tea—12 oz............ ......25-30 mg
Brewed coffee—8 oz.........................80-135 mg
Decaf coffee—8 oz.............................5 mg
Espresso—2oz..................................100 mg
Energy drink—8 oz............................80-300 mg

Keep in mind that cup size matters. You can get a 64-ounce soda from the fountain and Starbucks' smallest coffee size is a 12-ounce "Tall." There is always some wise guy who asserts "Tea has much more caffeine than coffee." I love this one because it is true BUT that is by weight only, not serving. One uses much less tea to brew a cup, so it actually has less caffeine by serving than coffee.

There is however, caffeine hidden away in many of the foods we love, foods that appear innocent.

Coffee ice cream has between 30 to 50 grams of caffeine, certainly enough to keep you up at night if you are sensitive. Caffeine lurks in some noncola sodas as well. Sunkist orange soda, for instance, has 41 milligrams per 12-ounce serving, almost as much as Mountain Dew at 52 grams. Carnation instant breakfast has 9 grams of caffeine, and so does a cup of hot chocolate. Some over-the-counter painkillers include caffeine, as well; Excedrin contains 132 grams per two-tablet dose, and maximum-strength Anacin lists 62.

❧

I'd rather take coffee than compliments just now.

. . . .

Louisa May Alcott, Little Women

Chapter 13

A Good Night's Sleep

. . . .

I mentioned earlier how my Grandfather used to get out of bed if he couldn't sleep and fix himself a nice cup of instant coffee to get himself back to dreamland. It worked for him, but he had an ironclad constitution. He often ate a half-pound of chocolate-covered peanuts right before dinner without dulling his appetite or causing him to gain weight, so maybe he was just weird.

The caffeine in coffee can certainly disrupt sleep. As a stimulant, it makes us feel more alert but it really cannot replace sleep. It functions by temporarily blocking the sleep inducing chemicals in the brain and increasing adrenaline production. Entering the bloodstream through the stomach and small intestine, caffeine takes effect within fifteen minutes of ingestion. Six hours must pass before half the caffeine from one cup of coffee wears off, and the balance may remain in the system for hours more.

There is no nutritional need at all for coffee or caffeine in the body, although the habitual coffee user may beg to differ, for the body soon becomes accustomed to its daily fix. Without it, the coffee drinker is left feeling sluggardly and listless.

The National Sleep Foundation notes that three cups of coffee per day is what they consider "moderate" consumption, while six or more cups a day is "excessive." (It depends on who you ask what is considered "moderate." The Alzheimer's Institute considers four to five cups a day to be moderate

71

consumption) They make the very sensible recommendation to "avoid caffeine near bedtime" to facilitate a good night's sleep. Raise your hand if this is news to you.

Caffeine interferes with the balance between stimulation and sedation by preventing "cool out" messages from getting to their destination in the brain. This shifts the whole nervous system into a higher gear and explains the better mental and athletic performance while caffeine is in the system.

Once the blocking of the body's adenosine receptors sets the new gear, the body reacts by creating more adenosine and more receptors and, voila! The previous balance is restored, and you need yet another cup of coffee to create the lift you crave—or just to keep your eyes open.

Drink enough coffee on a regular basis and the cycle whips around so quickly that it makes you sleepy! So, my grandfather was not a freak, just a man who enjoyed an excessive amount of coffee each day.

At a time in my life when I needed to rise at 4:00 a.m. daily in order to keep my business on track, the house presentable, and the kids fed, I drank excessive amounts of coffee in an attempt to keep moving. (I do not believe I was much of a treat to live with in those days.) When I started making a fourth pot of coffee around 3:00 p.m. every day, I decided it was not working anymore anyway, so I went cold turkey.

After a rotten few days of withdrawal, blinding headaches, and fuzzy head, I could see how truly exhausted I was without added stimulation in my system. Years of four or five hours of sleep a night had left me depleted in physical and emotional strength. With the caffeine out of my system, I didn't have the energy to mash a gnat. Because I had no choice at this point,

I caught up on my sleep, exercised more, and soon felt better. It was only when I added the correct amount of protein to my diet to keep my nutritional needs satisfied, that I could take up a more moderate coffee habit again, years later.

The variations in physical tolerance for caffeine are very real, and can change throughout a person's life due to nutritional and emotional stresses. On the other side of that coin is the 5 to10 percent of the population who are super sensitive to caffeine. I know of one naturopathic doctor who has always hated the smell and taste of coffee; she has never had even one cup of coffee in her life and has tested as allergic to it.

I now love my coffee, but really cannot manage more than two cups of espresso per morning. One very nice result of my restraint is that I can enjoy a rare cup in the evening and stay up way past my bedtime for something special, say, a night at the opera. I really need it then because although I am wildly fascinated by the spectacle and the music, if you put me in a dim room in a comfortable seat after 6:00 p.m., I tend to nod off. At $200 a pop for opera tickets, that is one expensive nap! I am grateful for the hours of enjoyment that my late night coffee gives me, but only every now and then.

Too Much Caffeine?

So, what's the deal with caffeine and coffee? Caffeine is considered both a benefit and drawback to coffee. Those who need an energy boost love the jumpstart they get from their treasured coffee break, but ironically find that the more they drink over time, the less of an effect they feel. One builds up a tolerance for caffeine over time, and then there is the devil to pay when you miss a cup or two—the dreaded caffeine-fiend withdrawal headache strikes.

A paradox in the coffee world is that the darker the roast, the less caffeine in the cup. Yep, espresso has less caffeine that Dunkin' regular. I am a big espresso fan, so this is good news for me. I can down my two shots per day without fretting about any untoward side effects.

Drinking decaf can feel less than satisfying to one accustomed to the high of high test, and the decaffeination process can itself be toxic. What's a coffee lover to do? Below you'll find the facts as we know them right now so you can navigate your way through a maze of Starbucks and Dunkin's to get what you need and what you want, and leave the everything else behind.

Decaffeination

There are three ways to get decaf from a cup of regular coffee, which contains an average of 180 to 200 grams of caffeine in an eight-ounce cup, according to the Mayo Clinic. Keep in mind that tests done daily on the same coffee order, same size, same type from the same coffeeshop once netted a 200-gram difference, and you will understand why getting an exact dose is a challenge.

Eighty percent of decaf coffee is decaffeinated via organic solvents like methylene chloride. The American Cancer Society has this on a list of human carcinogenics—not a recommended food group. The solvent is supposed to be removed from the beans, but residue is often found in coffee and tea decaffeinated with this method. Enough said; avoid it.

If your coffee label says it's "naturally decaffeinated," it was made using ethyl acetate, a chemical that occurs naturally in fruit. Because it occurs in fruit, which is safely consumed, the ethyl acetate is considered "natural." In this process, the beans are soaked in water. The water, which now contains the dissolved caffeine, is drawn off and mixed with ethyl acetate. It is then heated to evaporate the solvent and caffeine, then the water is returned to the beans, largely because it also supplies the coffee flavor. The solvent never actually touches the beans in this method, so is considered to be safe.

Another method uses CO_2 to dissolve the caffeine directly from the beans and the results are about the same as the water method—no toxic residue, but less flavor.

There was a time when carbon tetrachloride and formaldehyde were used to decaffeinate coffee, methods not looked upon with favor these days. Health hazards from your coffee should not be a concern if you watch for coffee with a label stating it was decaffeinated naturally or through the Swiss water process, according to Columbia University Health Services.

The water method leaves no toxic residue, but as it removes some of the flavor, sometimes less than stellar beans are mixed in, yielding an inferior-tasting cup. In addition, if beans of different regions are mixed, the flavors become muddied, resulting in a less precisely flavored coffee than one started with. In this method, after the water dissolves the caffeine, it is run through an activated-charcoal filter to remove the caffeine. The water is then mixed back in with the beans.

There are a few more reasons why decaf coffee is more expensive and less tasty. Beans destined to be decaf coffee have a few extra stamps on their passport. They must be chosen and sent to the decaf plant, processed in big batches, then shipped back. This explains why your favorite rare Sumatran blend may not be available sans caffeine.

The decaf beans are darker in color, which makes them a bit of a challenge to roast, for the roastary relies on color to know when the beans are done to a turn. So the dark decaf beans may not be roasted to the precise perfection as regular beans.

In the end, these beans usually spend less time in the roaster, so wind up with less of the subtle flavor notes that sophisticated coffee drinkers look for. Decaf drinkers, on the other hand, are used to drinking a smoother, blander cup than regular coffee drinkers. As demand rises for better organic decafs, so will the availability of these better brews. Keep on asking for the best!

Most decaf is made from Robusta beans because they have the strongest flavor, but Robusta is also very acidic. So look out for acid-related troubles if you drink lots of decaf in your effort to drown your sorrows over losing the caffeine. High acidic levels in coffee contribute to acid reflux, irritable-bowel syndrome, and some say, cardiovascular disease.

We think of caffeine as the culprit in making us jumpier, but studies show that other components of coffee that survive the decaffeination process can cause changes in the autonomic nervous system, raising the heart rate and stimulating the bowels, just like regular coffee. Damned if you do, damned if you don't.

In addition to all the above, switching to decaf has been shown to boost cholesterol production, as well as to cause an increase in rheumatoid arthritis. On the plus side, there are studies showing a benefit to those at risk for diabetes in drinking coffee of any kind, decaf or regular, with slightly better outcomes in the caffeinated test subjects. On the other hand, caffeinated coffee can increase blood pressure and may pose a health threat to people with cardiovascular disease, while decaffeinated coffee does not pose such a risk.

Decaf has to have, by law, 97 percent of the caffeine removed. Starbucks says their tall, 12-ounce coffee, which is their smallest size, contains 11 grams of caffeine. It would be good to remember if you keep getting refills, that the content, though small, can add up over a day of drinking.

Remember, decaf is not the same as caffeine free! Given that as small an amount as 10 milligrams of caffeine can be detected by changes in the body, which the drinker can easily perceive, one should take care in the amount of decaf consumed.

If coffee or tea is not your thing, and even the decaf versions keep you up, I can recommend Teeccino, a masterful blend of healthy ingredients that may be enjoyed day or night. Creator Caroline MacDougall, an award winning herbal designer, has been mixing herbal combinations for decades. Teechino, brews up just like coffee and comes in many enticing flavors.

Chapter 14

Cholesterol Concerns

. . . .

Some types of coffee can raise cholesterol levels. The Robusta bean, typically used in decaf coffee because of its strong flavor, can be a contributor to this effect. A study done at Baylor University found that cafestol, a compound found in coffee, elevates cholesterol by hijacking a receptor in an intestinal pathway critical to its regulation.

"Cafestol is the most potent dietary cholesterol-elevating agent known," said Dr. David Moore, professor of molecular and cellular biology at Baylor College of Medicine, and Dr. Marie-Louise Ricketts, a postdoctoral student and first author of the report. Decaffeinating coffee does not remove the cafestol. There is some good news, however; the cafestol can be removed by passing the coffee through a paper filter.

Competing studies show that coffee contains niacin, a substance found to reduce cholesterol levels and this is found equally in decaf and regular coffee. In fact, most of the health benefits of coffee are also present in decaf. Just remember, in a study covering twenty-four years of people drinking six cups of coffee per day, there was absolutely NO ill effect on their longevity. Enjoy your coffee and think happy thoughts!

Nancy Astor: "If I were your wife, I would put poison
in your coffee."
Sir Winston Churchill: "And if I were your husband,
I would drink it."

. . . .

Dialogue between Nancy Astor and
Sir Winston Churchill

Chapter 15

Coffee Tips and Tricks

I use a Nespresso coffee maker that brews an excellent cup with a thick crema on top. The coffee comes in individual pods that are easy to use and, even though they seem a bit pricy, there is absolutely no waste. I drink up every last drop, it is so delicious. Nespresso chooses from the top three percent of specialty coffees grown around the world and comes in a dazzling variety of flavors, both regular and decaf.

When the cup is so rich and satisfying, I feel no need to overdo it; perfect satisfaction comes my way every morning! Half the fun is anticipation, so I drink a few cups of jasmine tea and some ice water before I even get out of bed. (I keep an electric kettle and thermal water carafe on the bedside table.) By the time I make my way down to the espresso machine, I am hydrated and ready to enjoy my first cup of coffee.

Look for fair trade and organic coffee. It is better for you and will encourage a more sustainable industry which will result in better coffee and more delicious varieties for you to choose. Seek out local small batch roasteries for the best of the best.

Use a filter pot if cholesteral is a concern, for this method of brewing can reduce bad cholesteral. If you love coffee but it doesn't love you, then try a low acid coffee to see if that helps your digestive difficulties.

Chocolate

Make a list of important things to do today. At the top of your list, put "eat chocolate." Now, you'll get at least one thing done today.

Gina Hayes

Chapter 16

The Long Way Around to Chocolate

· ·

In 1966 I took a trip to Switzerland that subtly changed the direction of my life. As an adventurous sixteen-year-old, I was so eager to join my French class on this summer excursion that I pulled out all the stops trying to persuade my parents to spring for what was, at that time, a huge sum, so I could "go abroad." In the end, I got my best friend, Katie, turned on to the idea.

Katie attended a neighboring high school, the new one in town that had a swimming pool and air conditioning. If you think that wouldn't, or maybe shouldn't, matter to young scholars, it's certain that you never sweated your way through endless hours of tedious classes in a sweltering northern Virginia spring or fall.

My high school was newly built as well—schools were popping up all over town to handle the influx of baby-boom teens, and tax-rich Fairfax County had money to burn for the designing and building of such edifices. Thomas A. Edison was an undistinguished brick pile with the usual pale-green and buff tile walls, giant cafeteria, spectacular auditorium, and manual arts wing. We did have our very own special feature—a planetarium. Bet your high school didn't have one! But we surely would have chosen air conditioning over the planetarium, had we been offered the choice.

This was the era of school tracking. Your fate was decided in elementary school, where you were slotted into one track or another. If you showed promise handling your Big Mo pencil as a second grader, clever kid—academic track for you! Good grades and college were expected of you and if you did not live up to those expectations, well, you could expect meeting with guidance counselors, extra credit work, summer school, and stern lectures about "not living up to your potential."

Not so stellar in third grade reading group? You joined the "looking at pictures" set, where, perhaps, if you were a girl, you could train to be a secretary, or learn to repair trucks, if you were a boy—no need to waste a college prep class on you. I knew this at the time because a dastardly second grade teacher labeled my active imagination as "daydreaming" (what a crime for a six-year-old!) and put me in that "looking at pictures" group. A kind and dedicated third grade teacher, on assessing her new charges, felt I had been badly used and came in early every morning to give me extra tutoring so I could join my rightful place among the fast trackers.

Like most kids, I did not respond well to my allotted groove, whichever one it was. Destined for college (but learn to type, just in case you need a job as a secretary, to fall back on), I loved reading Hamlet, excelled at biology, was a big dummy in algebra class, and insisted on taking drafting, engineering, and wood shop. I would have ventured into the electronics wing, but it was pretty far down the "boy's hall." Prudence, plus some truly horrifying experiences with the fellas in wood shop, kept me back. That is a tale for another day (see my upcoming book, *Sorry, So Sorry: Letters of Apology I Should Have Received, but Never Did, So I Wrote Them Myself.*)

I loved the idea of speaking French and traveling the world as a sophisticated woman of mystery. Mystery, because I couldn't boil down my diverse ambitions to a single profession.

"Astronaut" was as close as I came to declaring a career path, but when I found out I would have to join the military, excel at math and, well, deal with all those boys, I made a quick switch to a career in the arts.

Plunging into a Great Society-funded art school over summer vacation, I switched all my elective classes to art the following year. I was raring to go to Paris, starve in a garret, and paint passionately. One small problem was my decidedly poor performance in the six years of French classes I had already taken.

Advancing only so far as French three, I could not in good conscience blame my record on the weak start provided by the redheaded Marborough sisters in middle school. These teachers were identical twins, one of whom taught regularly, with the other substituting as needed. We never really figured out who was who, but one thing was glaringly obvious: neither had a clue about pronouncing French words as the French do. They each boasted an extreme southern (that's United States southern,) accent.

Even to the completely untutored ear, the sounds coming out of their brightly lipsticked mouths did not resemble any French we had ever heard. Granted, most of us were basing our judgment on Pepé Le Pew cartoons, but still . . . We mimicked and mouthed the words, knowing all along we would be laughed out of any French venue where we might test our newly acquired linguistic skills.

As I say, I can't blame the Marboroughs, for my high school French teacher was demure, patient, and possessed of an excellent accent and a sense of style as fine as any any Frenchwoman's. I guess it was another case of not living up to my potential, failing to apply myself, etc., etc.

My plot was to fix it all with a summer in Switzerland. Studying French was essential to my life plan to become (somehow simultaneously) a starving artist driven by my creative vision, and a rich and famous woman of the world. I figured I could work out the details later. Now I just wanted out of a blistering summer in Alexandria with nothing much to do, except the summer school class in geometry I was being urged to consider.

Katie was eager to join me in the adventure and we set out to persuade our parents. Because she didn't know any of the other kids who had signed up, Katie wanted to go only if I came along. Her alliance turned out to be my ace in the hole. My parents steadfastly refused to go into debt for my summer of dubious study, until my friend's mom managed to convince them.

A top student, Katie Beacher could always use another star on her glowing academic record, and maybe her mom knew how much we longed and needed to expand our world beyond the small town atmosphere we enjoyed at home. Whatever her reasons, I will always be grateful she helped make that dream come true.

Mrs. Beacher had, after all, treated us to our first fancy restaurant meal, having demonstrated how to order, which fork to use, and how to tip. After our indoctrination, she left us on our own in a swank restaurant while she attended a business meeting, thus imparting another vital bit of information about grown-up life: a woman can (and must) compete and win in the world of business. She provided a powerful example.

With the style, grace, and fierceness of the true southern woman, she passed along the wisdom of the generations and gave us a good, long peek behind the veil, showing us how much work went into sophisticated, serene, and seemingly effortless southern charm. Charm that worked its magic on my folks.

So we triumphed and the trip was on. Excitement built as we packed and prepared for a trip that was a to be pivotal point in my life. Thank you, Mom and Dad, for givng in and paying my way.

The visit to Europe gave me more than a summer getaway, and the dubious progress I made in French. It gave me a new orientation for pleasure, one I embraced, with never a glance back to my Puritan roots.

When you think of Switzerland, you think of chocolate—well, I do—and I was eager to make the most of my short stay. Discovering that Swiss chocolate bars were much larger than the ones at home and that they came in a huge variety of types and flavors was a wonderful surprise.

At the time, I had seen only the usual milk chocolate Hershey and Mars bars in the grocery store checkout line. Those, along with Sky Bars and the ubiquitous Christmas Whitman's Sampler, had provided my only experience with chocolate, and while I loved it dearly in those forms, it was old news. Spending my Swiss francs on a giant, exotic Swiss chocolate bar every day was an indulgence I felt entitled to, as I was not sure when such a chance might come again.

I was on the receiving end of all manner of cautions and raised eyebrows from my peers because of my chocolate obsession. As a teenaged girl in the mid sixties, I was well aware that much depended on keeping my figure. Despite downing a huge bar of chocolate all by myself every day, I actually lost weight on that trip. Eat your heart out, peers.

Mind you, we weren't couch potatoes. Every day, we climbed the steep hills of Montreaux and walked miles around the lake, so my activity level was pretty high. Nevertheless, it was a nice surprise to come home a little slimmer and stronger. Nor were the predicted pimples and acne a problem. My skin was as clear as before my chocolate binge began. I was quite pleased with myself for foiling the naysayers and enjoying myself freely.

Turns out there is a scientific explanation for all that, as I found when researching this book. So, bring on the chocolate, it's back to the future for me, as I munch on my giant bar and set out for a midafternoon break on a very different shore from the one I walked around that summer, forty-plus years ago at Lake Geneva.

Chocolate is not only one of life's great pleasures, it can be astoundingly good for you, but dosage is critical. Too much of a good thing can be very bad for you, indeed.

In the following chapters, you'll find a rundown on the beneficial effects of chocolate for prevention and cure of various ills that plague man and woman-kind, not the least of which is depression. There is nothing so soothing, nothing so directly brightening to the disposition, as chocolate.

I hope you'll find a place in your health routine for a nibble of sweet reward. Read on to discover the secrets of chocolate. Be sure to indulge as you read, and buy another book for your skeptical friends when they give you the stink eye for enjoying yourself. They're just envious.

Now excuse me while I go to the store. I seem to have run out of Cadbury's—or was it Lindt?

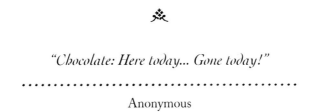

"Chocolate: Here today... Gone today!"

....

Anonymous

Chapter 17

The History of Chocolate

. . . .

How long have humans been craving their chocolate fix? Quite a while it seems. Modern folk are not alone in believing the taste of chocolate to be divine; Aztecs and Mayans thought the cacao bean had magical properties and used it in sacred rituals. It was also used as currency, and a tax of beans was collected on landholders. The Mayans used cocao beans as early as 600 BC. Anthropologists from the University of Pennsylvania dated cocoa residue on pottery shards as far back as 1400 BC when it was consumed as an alcoholic beverage.

Just to give you a bit of a timeline: during that same era, Thebes, the capitol of Egypt, was the largest city in the world; Moses fled Egypt; the temples at Luxor began to be built; and the Iron Age got under way in Asia and India.

Christopher Columbus, the first European to discover chocolate, dismissed his discovery as irrelevant to his goal of finding a passage to India. He left town without ever grasping the signifigance of the beans that were used as currency and to make a sacred (and delicious) beverage.

The Spanish had to wait for chocolate until Hernando Cortés to come along, twenty years later. He got it right, presumably because he hired himself an interpreter. Cortés recognized the value of the strange beans and brought some back to Europe. Sugar was added to chocolate and soon everyone was drinking it—everyone who could afford it, that is. The beverage was believed to have medicinal properties; even better, it was thought to be an aphrodisiac and was apparently a favorite of that famous lover, Casanova.

The shipping and lengthy preparation of the cacoa beans made it an expensive drink only the wealthy could enjoy, until the steam engine brought the price down by mechanizing the processing. In the early 1800s, a Dutch chemist, Johannes van Houten, patented a press that removed the cocoa butter from the nibs. He thus created powdered cocoa and, by adding alkaline salts to cut the bitter flavor, produced Dutch cocoa.

The very first chocolate candy bar was created in 1847 by Joseph Fry, an Englishman, who put the cocoa butter back into the Dutched cocoa, added sugar, and cast the resulting paste into a mold. Two years later, John Cadbury began selling candy bars and boxes of chocolate candies in England and in 1919 the two companies merged and continue to made chocolate under the name Cadbury's.

This was all dark chocolate, until around 1880, when Daniel Peter of Switzerland, a former candle manufacturer who had fallen on hard times after the rise of the oil lamp, experimented until he was able to successfully combine milk with chocolate. The milk he used to make the solid chocolate was a dehydraded version of condensed milk made by the his neighbor Henri Nestle, a manufacturer of condensed milk. The two later merged as the Nestle company.

In 1900 Milton Hershey developed his own technique for adding milk to chocolate, creating a candy bar with good shelf life. He set up his plant in rural Pennsylvania, close to the milk supply, in a little town that would be renamed Hershey.

Today chocolate is a twenty billion dollar business in the US and close to one hundred billion worldwide. Each American eats about half a pound a month. If that were all dark chocolate, it would be just about the right amount to protect their health from hypertension, cardiovascular disease, and diabetes, for chocolate does indeed, as the ancients believed, have medicinal uses, lightening mood and improving cardiovascular health.

If you have not already located some delicious dark chocolate, may I suggest you give into your craving and munch while reading the next bit. Chocolate is available in many types. Varying the quantities of the different ingredients produces different forms and flavors of chocolate. Other flavors can be obtained by varying the time and temperature when roasting the beans.

Unsweetened chocolate, also known as bitter, baking chocolate, or cooking chocolate, is pure chocolate liquor mixed with some form of fat to produce a solid substance. The pure, ground, roasted cocoa beans impart a strong, deep chocolate flavor. With the addition of sugar it is used as the base for cakes, brownies, confections, and cookies.

Dark chocolate is produced by adding fat and sugar to cocoa. It is chocolate with little or no milk. The US has no official definition for dark chocolate, including it in the range classified as sweet chocolate, but European rules specify a minimum of 35 percent cocoa solids. Many chocolate products are sold as dark chocolate however and it can be confusing to choose the most healthful.

I have seen chocolate bars labeled with the percentage of dark chocolate, ranging from 35 percent to 90 percent. There is no way of knowing the actual antioxident count in your chosen brand so without getting bogged down in these challenges, delicious though they may be, I suggest choosing the highest percentage dark chocolate you can happily enjoy.

Milk chocolate contains cocoa solids, milk and sugar. Milk chocolates are typically much sweeter than dark chocolate and many popular candy bars that are chocolate based use milk chocolate.

Once you have your chocolate fix in hand, you might not care how it got there. On the other hand (the one holding this book), perhaps your awareness has been heightened by indulging, and you may be interested in knowing a few details about your chocolate's journey.

It began as a cocao bean in a pod on a cacao tree in the shady tropical rainforest near the equator. The shady forest floor provides a perfect environment for the young cacao tree, but the rush to produce more cocao beans has resulted in cutting down the forest to provide an environment of full sun, because cacao trees grown in full sun create a bigger crop. However, they live for only ten years, leaving a region without its rainforest, with depleted soil, and no cash crop to show for it. A tree grown in the traditional manner will not have so big a crop, but will grow and produce for up to twenty-five years. As the rainforest disappears, the climate changes caused by deforestation result in further reduction in yield.

When a crop is grown all by itself as a monoculture, it is a sitting duck for pests and blight. More pesticides must be used, marring the healthful quality and purity of the final product. As the rain forests diminish, new techniques and locations are being sought to satisfy the growing demand for chocolate worldwide.

Sustainable cacao farms are supported by the Rainforest Alliance, which certifies cocoa as being grown in a sustainable manner. Cacao is farmed on over 18 million acres of land and provides a livelihood for over 40 million people. The Rainforest

Alliance partners with agencies in cacao-growing countries to support, encourage and legislate sustainable shade grown plants. It is those plants that produce the cocao beans for the chocolate we can enjoy guilt free.

Cocao beans are similar in size and shape to almonds, growing inside cocao pods. The hard cocao pod is about the size of a Nerf football. It grows off the branches and trunk of the cocao tree and each pod contains between thirty to forty beans.

Once the mature cacao is harvested, which must be done by hand as the pods mature at different times, beans are removed from the pods and fermented for two to eight days. The fermented beans are then dried. Next they are sorted by type and roasted.

There is an art to this roasting and the quality of the final product owes much to the care given to this process. After roasting, the beans are transfered to a winnower that separates out the shells and leaves the nibs, as the beans are now called. (You can buy the cocao bean hulls in bags as mulch for a heavenly smelling garden, especially when it rains.) The nibs, somewhat chocolaty, but bitter, are now ready for processing.

The conching machine, first invented by Rodolphe Lindt in 1879, comewhat resembled a chonch shell. In it, the nibs are slightly heated and ground, reducing them to a viscous liquid called liquor (no alcohol, sorry) which has a high fat content from the cocoa butter. The process which varies in length from six to seventy two hours, releases flavors and creates a smooth final product. If this refining step is ommited, the chocolate will be grainy.

The warm liquid, after conching, is pumped into kettles where it is heated and cooled, a process called tempering, which gives the chocolate its characteristic silky texture and glossy surface. It is then cast into molds, where a little shaking removes air bubbles, and a candy bar is born, ready to be wrapped and shipped to your local shop.

The art of making fine chocolate depends on the environment where the cacao is grown, the care taken in harvesting, the proper fermenting, drying, roasting, conching and tempering. The variables give us a broad variety of quality and flavors from which to choose.

Shade-grown cocoa is better for the environment, better for the people who work on the cocoa farms, and more sustainable than sun grown cocoa. Free from contaminants, pesticides, and herbicides, it is better for you as well. For this reason, I seek out sources of this high quality chocolate and support its continued production with my dollars.

One such company is Sibu Sura Chocolates, whose founder, Julie McLean, forges relationships with bean growers in Peru, procuring the finest beans for her products. The effort pays off, for their single origin bean, 100% organic, fair trade certified chocolates are some of the finest I've tasted. You can find out more about the chocolate and their intriguing name at the web site www.sibusura.com.

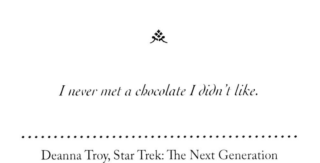

I never met a chocolate I didn't like.

....

Deanna Troy, Star Trek: The Next Generation

.

Chapter 18

Can Chocolate Really Be Good For You?

. . . .

You may have seen the good news about chocolate, touting the newly discovered health benefits. Here is a sampling:

- Eating chocolate while pregnant causes your babies to smile and laugh more!
- Does chocolate make you clever?
- Chocolate improves mental function in the elderly.
- Heart attacks prevented by a daily dose of chocolate.
- Chocolate prevents tooth decay.
- Chocolate: the more you eat, the better you feel!
- Chocolate soon to be declared a "health food" in Europe.

I am not too sure about the babies smiling, but if mom is happy, everybody has a better chance of being happy, so, yeah, I'll go along. Read on to learn about the science behind these headlines and rejoice, for there is truth in them all!

Chocolate in its pure form is full of concentrated antioxidants called polyphenols. Some types of polyphenols are called flavonoids and tannins. In the human body, these substances have many documented beneficial effects.

Chocolate is an antihypertensive and can be used to control high blood pressure. As an antithrombotic it is useful to thin the blood and keep the arteries clear. Tannins have an antibacterial effect and can interfere with the action of bacteria on teeth.

Who knew that chocolate could decrease your chance of tooth decay! You know that sugar has the opposite effect, of course. And it's unlikely that you'd get carried away brushing your teeth with unsweetened chocolate as the taste is not pleasant.

The metabolic effects of chocolate are being researched, but it appears that adding dark chocolate to the diet does not promote weight gain (or loss, it should be noted) but does improve health by thinning the blood, dissolving clots, lowering blood pressure, and strengthening the heart muscle.

The effects of certain concentrated antioxidant substances on the SIRT1 gene, one of the genes that regulate longevity, has been proven in recent studies. This is complex stuff which is often and mistakenly boiled down to fascinating, compelling "news" that has no factual basis.

Chocolate is not a miracle, but as a form of treatment or prevention for a host of ills, is surprisingly effective. There is no evidence that it will make you live 150 years; you can't eat unlimited chocolate and become sleek and gorgeous; it will not counteract years of poor dietary choices or genes that make you more susceptible to heart disease. Nevertheless, if taken in the right amounts, chocolate can help with all of the above.

If you can head off heart disease, the nation's number one killer, you increase your lifespan. If you can make your life a little more content by adding in a pleasure or two, you might also enjoy your longer life a little bit more. Please do remember that increasing your intake of polyphenols, flavonoids, and tannins contributes to overall health only if not taken with a corresponding increase in dietary sugar and fat.

This chart gives you an idea which chocolate is better for you. Hint: it's all about the antioxidants, the content of which varies according to type. A good rule of thumb is the darker, the better. The FDA has no definition of dark chocolate and percentage of cocoa varies greatly, so these are guidelines, not facts. I am using the term dark chocolate to cover a range of sweetened chocolate that contains no signifigant milk content and averaging the very dark and not so dark. The following information comes from a study done by the Department of Nutrition and Dietetics, Faculty of Medicine and Health Sciences, Universiti Putra Malaysia and reported in the journal *Molecules* in 2009.

The report states "The polyphenol content in chocolates varies greatly depending on processing techniques such as fermentation of cocoa beans and alkalinization of cocoa powders," so please consider the following information a guide to the relative merits rather than the gospel.

Type of Chocolate	Phenolics	Flavinoids
Dark Chocolate	579 mg	28 mg
Milk Chocolate	160 mg	13 mg
White Chocolate	126 mg	8 mg

Cooking or Baking Chocolate is unsweetened and has 70 to 99 percent solid cocoa. Did you ever sneak a taste when your mom was making a cake? I did, and it was indeed bitter. Without the sugar to balance it out, the taste is chalky and unpleasant. One ounce of cooking chocolate is equal to three tablespoons of cocoa powder plus one tablespoon of butter or oil.

Dark Chocolate contains a minimum of 35 percent solid cocoa in its popular form as a chocolate bar or semisweet chips, (this is the european standard, the United States has no such required cocoa content) with fat and sugar and very little milk. As dark chocolate is a term used frequently in the studies I site and as it is a familiar term to most chocolate lovers, I use it in this book even though "dark chocolate" has no official definition in the US.

We all know the reputation of fat and sugar; there is all too much of it lurking in foods we eat every day, so it must be carefully monitored. Fat has recently enjoyed better press, as it is needed to process many fat-soluble vitamins, so possibly should not be severely restricted.

Milk Chocolate has comparatively little polyphenol and flavonoid content compared with dark chocolate (about a third) and much more fat and sugar. This gives it a delicious mouth feel, and mild taste, but rather reduces its efficacy as a source of health building antioxidants, creating instead an opportunity to add pounds.

White Chocolate is chocolate with the cocoa removed, making it pretty much devoid of positive antioxidant qualities. I use it for decoration and pack the cocoa in wherever I can to get best bang for my buck, chocolate-wise.

To get an extra 600 milligrams of antioxidents (polyphenols and flavinoids combined) from dark chocolate alone, one would need to consume about 100 grams. That is three and a half ounces of dark chocolate or three tablespoons of cocoa per day. One of these extra big chocolate bars is about three to three and a half ounces, so that's a lot of chocolate, sugar and fat! But wait! You can do better; just read the labels carefully.

Here is my rather unscientific method of justifying more chocolate in my life. The amount of cocoa solids needed to be considered "dark chocolate" is a mere 35 percent. The label on my dark chocolate bar from Whole Foods says it has 56 percent cocoa solids, so I can eat a little more than half a bar and still get my 600 milligrams of polyphenols. That comes to about seven grams of fat and 275 calories. In fact, the serving size indicated on the package is half a bar. Okay, I can live with that.

The American Dental Society recommends if you are going to eat chocolate on a regular basis, to eat it all at once, then brush your teeth. I personally like to spread my treats throughout the day, but I am passing along their advice to you all the same. I also drink a lot of plain water, so that may be sparing my teeth. Go ahead and resolve to indulge regularly—it could be the healthiest thing you do all year!

Strength is the ability to break a chocolate bar into four pieces with your bare hands - and then eat just one of those pieces.

· ·

Judith Viorst

Chapter 19

Hearts and Chocolate

. . . .

Cardiovascular disease is the leading cause of death worldwide. Even a small improvement in the heart health of the population will translate into thousands of lives saved and much suffering eased. Could a daily bite of chocolate really benefit your heart? When the treatment is this easy to take, who wouldn't want to fight heart disease?

Before adding in any new treatments—if you can call chocolate a treatment—modifying your existing diet seems a sensible first step. Even if one is genetically predisposed towards cardiovascular disease, a healthy diet rich in polyphenols and flavonoids can make a real difference in outcomes. Sources for polyphenols in the American diet are highly colored fruits and vegetables, tea, wine, and chocolate. Cocoa products contain the highest concentrate of these antioxidants.

In a broad-reaching study of studies (meta study), Harvard University researchers Eric L. Ding, Susan M. Hutfless, Xin Ding, and Saket Girotra, took a close look at previous studies from around the world as to the effect of flavonoid- and polyphenol-rich dark chocolate consumption on cardiovascular disease. This Harvard meta study, which reviewed 136 previous studies from 1956 to 2005, concluded a positive benefit from consumption of dark chocolate and revealed the possibility that the milk in milk chocolate might inhibit the absorption of flavonoids, making that form of chocolate a poor choice for boosting antioxidant levels.

113

In another study, researchers from the Cardiovascular Epidemiology Research Unit, Department of Medicine, Beth Israel Deaconess Medical Center, Harvard Medical School in Boston, Massachusetts, investigated the effect of chocolate consumption on death from heart failure in middle-aged to elderly women. They followed 31,823 women aged forty-eight to eighty-three years old from 1998 to 2006.

They concluded that "In this population, moderate habitual chocolate intake was associated with a lower rate of heart failure, hospitalization or death." They noted that the chocolate consumption had to exceed a minimum daily intake (one serving a day, which is about half a big candy bar or 1.75 ounces) to give results and that occasional chocolate use did not yield significant results.

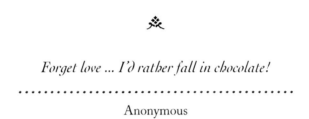

Forget love ... I'd rather fall in chocolate!

Anonymous

Chapter 20

Chocolate and Inflammation

· ·

Lifestyle triggers for heart disease are widely known: smoking, stress, obesity, and low activity level can cause inflammation of the walls of the arteries that serve the heart. Inflammation is the body's natural response to these negative stimuli. The immune system sends in the troops of white blood cells in an attempt to repair the damage and control the inflammation. The white blood cells adhere to artery walls blocking the blood flow and causing heart failure.

Decreasing inflammation can have a positive effect on heart disease, high blood pressure, and even cancer, so naturally, one would want to stop smoking, eat a healthy diet, loose weight if overweight, and get some exercise. The addition of cocoa to the diet has been shown to decrease inflammation and increase brachial artery blood flow.

In a study designed to test the effectiveness of dark chocolate on cholesterol levels, Penn State researchers showed that chocolate doesn't just lower your levels of LDL cholesterol; it also slows the rate at which LDL oxidizes. The oxidation of LDL in cholesterol is believed to play a key role in the hardening of arteries. Slowing this oxidation may actually slow the development and progression of heart disease. This study was published in the *American Journal of Clinical Nutrition.*

There you have it. Eating a modest amounts of dark chocolate daily can support heart health and even may reverse some conditions. Remember that the effective dose is one or two ounces of dark chocolate, not milk chocolate! Don't get hung up on the percent of cacoa or exactly how dark your chocolate is, but do choose high-quality dark chocolate that is from shade-grown trees, if possible, to get the highest levels of polyphenols for your buck.

Nine out of ten people like chocolate.
The tenth person always lies.

• •

John Q. Tullius

Chapter 21

Chocolate and Hypertension

. . . .

High blood pressure—hypertension—is called the silent killer because there are typically no symptoms of this condition. When the force of blood on artery walls as it makes its circuit through the body is too great, damage to your heart, brain, arteries, and kidneys is the result. About one in three adults in the US has high blood pressure.

High blood pressure causes hardening and thickening of the arteries and may lead to heart attack, stroke, kidney damage, and loss of vision. This condition often has no symptoms before damage is done, so monitoring blood pressure is done as part of just about every encounter we have with a medical professional.

Uncontrolled high blood pressure also interferes with the ability to think clearly. Trouble with memory and understanding concepts is more common in people with high blood pressure. The longer this condition persists, the greater the damage, and it becomes a problem for a great many people as they age.

In men, high blood pressure causes trouble with sexual performance. Unfortunately, the medication for reducing high blood pressure can cause similar symptoms, which leads to a problem with patients' following doctor's orders and taking the prescription.

As obesity is a leading cause of high blood pressure, why add chocolate to the diets of patients who are already obese? In a study that concluded in 2012 the Australian Diabetes, Obesity and Lifestyle study researchers found that of the 2013 participants with hypertension, with no history of cardiovascular disease and not receiving antihypertensive therapy, those who consumed dark chocolate with a polyphenol content of 500-plus milligrams, significantly reduced both total cholesterol and low-density lipoprotein-cholesterol levels.

The blood pressure and cholesterol-lowering properties associated with dark chocolate consumption could potentially prevent seventy nonfatal cardiovascular events and fifteen cardiovascular-related deaths per 10,000 population annually.

Assuming that $42 is spent per person per year on a dark chocolate consumption per patient, the strategy would be cost effective. Considering that cardiovascular disease is the leading cause of death worldwide, a small investment in "the food of the Gods" could pay off very well. The study also concluded that "Chocolate benefits from being, by and large, a pleasant and hence sustainable treatment option." Indeed!

Many studies find that cocoa-rich foods could alleviate high blood pressure in test subjects. Pooling the results of several previous studies a team of researchers from Melbourne, Australia, curious about the role of dark chocolate in heart health, looked at twenty studies in which adults ate dark chocolate or cocoa. More than 850 people participated in the trials that generally ran from two to eight weeks.

Consuming dark chocolate reduced the blood pressure of test subjects who already had high blood pressure, but not on those who had pressure in the normal range. They also discovered that blood pressure did not drop below normal, even when very high amounts of polyphenol chocolate were consumed. In addition, the higher the polyphenol content the more pronounced was the effect of normalizing blood pressure. How amazing—chocolate seems to be profoundly on our side when it comes to regulating blood pressure.

Since even small reductions in blood pressure substantially reduce cardiovascular risk, it would seem that including dark chocolate in their diet might be a good move for those who suffer high blood pressure. It certainly poses no risk for those with normal blood pressure. The study concluded "Current guidelines strongly recommend integration of lifestyle modification and complementary treatment with the use of conventional blood pressure medications."

If you have high blood pressure, don't stop taking your medication, but try adding dark chocolate to your diet and perhaps you can reduce the dose of your medication. Be sure to have your doctor do the monitoring, as self-prescribing can prove dangerous!

It has been shown as proof positive that carefully prepared chocolate is as healthful a food as it is pleasant; that it is nourishing and easily digested... that it is above all helpful to people who must do a great deal of mental work.

Anthelme Brillat-Savarin

Chapter 22

Chocolate and Diabetes

· ·

About a fifth of the world's population has some form of metabolic syndrome including type 2 diabetes, which has been on the rise in the US and 175 countries worldwide over the last 10 years. It is especially alarming that type 2 diabetes is showing up in children.

In type 2 diabetes, the body does not produce enough insulin or the pancreas does not properly process the insulin. Insulin, the hormone that helps cells make use of glucose, sucrose, and starch in your body, breaks down these nutrients from your food.

The rise in diabetes is often attributed to high-fructose-sweetened drinks, both because of their popularity and increasing size. High-fructose corn syrup, although it is metabolized by the body in the same way as other types of sugars, has a few additional complications. Certain "satisfaction" levels may not be reached after consuming high-fructose corn syrup, thus leaving the body craving even more sugary treats.

I don't know about you, but I need very little encouragement in craving sweets, so I avoid high-fructose corn-syrup-sweetened foods. This is not an easy task as the sweetener is found in just about every processed food from cookies, where you may expect to find it, to ketchup and salad dressing, where you may not expect it.

In a study published online (November 27, 2012,) in *Global Public Health* covering adults over age twenty from 199 countries, researchers examined the relationship between the prevalence of diabetes and body mass index, also considering the types of food most often consumed in each country. They also noted whether there was a high consumption of high-fructose corn syrup. Findings indicated a correlation between the incidence of diabetes and high-fructose consumption.

The countries with the lowest HFCS consumption levels were Australia, China, Denmark, France, the UK, and Uruguay, which showed an average percentage of the population with diabetes at 6.7 percent. The US by contrast was the biggest user of HFCS, at about fifty-five pounds of the stuff per person per year. The high consumption countries, including the US, Hungary, Slovakia, Canada, Bulgaria, Argentina, Korea, Japan and Mexico, had a 20 percent higher incidence of type 2 diabetes.

The prevalence of cardiometabolic disorders places a big burden on society, not to mention the suffering endured by those with these diseases. The World Health Organization notes that these disorders are largely preventable. Diet is the key lifestyle factor in getting diabetes, a factor that can be modified for prevention.

In a study comparing the results of previous research and examining it for clues to the best direction for dietary recommendations, researchers at the University of Cambridge, Strangeways Research Laboratory, Cambridge, UK evaluated the association between chocolate consumption and cardiometabolic disorders in adults. The study gave more weight or credence to reports of chocolate consumption that were validated as opposed to self-reported. No fudging was allowed (couldn't resist), and adjustments were made for weight, age, smoking, gender, and body mass.

They evaluated high and low chocolate consumption and also took into account the polyphenol content of the chocolate type consumed—white, milk, or dark—and concluded that "Five of the seven studies reported a beneficial association between higher levels of chocolate consumption and the risk of cardiometabolic disorders." and they added, "The highest levels of chocolate consumption were associated with a 37 percent reduction in cardiovascular incidents and a twenty-nine percent reduction in stroke compared with the lowest levels of chocolate consumed."

My conclusion is that adding dark chocolate to your daily diet will keep your heartbeat strong, your metabolism functioning well, your blood sugars in balance, and your mood upbeat.

Chapter 23

Chocolate and Obesity

. . . .

It's all well and good to extol the health virtues of a regular chocolate habit, but won't all that chocolate make me fat? Nope, not really. New research shows that people who eat chocolate tend to be thinner than the population of abstainers.

A study of 1,000 people done at the University of California at San Diego, showed that people who ate chocolate regularly—several times a week, rather than occasionally—were thinner than those who seldom ate it. How often you eat chocolate, rather than the quantity seems to be an indicator of slimness.

Lead author of the study, Dr. Beatrice Golomb, said, "Our findings appear to add to a body of information suggesting that the composition of calories, not just the number of them, matters for determining their ultimate impact on weight." To put this into a visual for you: Dr. Golomb cited that a 120-pound, five-foot-tall woman was likely to weigh five pounds less if she ate chocolate five times a week. Pass the truffles please!

Dr. Golomb cited other studies showing that antioxidant compounds called catechins improve lean muscle function and reduce weight. These studies were done on rodents, but still. I am a believer after my teen summer in Switzerland, where I ate a three-ounce bar daily and lost weight. That's a pound and a third a week, five and a quarter pounds a month. My mood was pretty darn good, too, come to think of it.

I remember back in the early days of "health food" when Adele Davis was a popular authority on diet and supplements. She maintained that one should not focus on weight loss, but rather on building health. Good advice, I think, as the former creates a culture of denial and lack, and the latter, one of abundance and positivity.

I believe that chocolate—dark chocolate—when eaten regularly and with a modicum of restraint, will contribute to a healthy weight and a satisfied life. And that's backed up by the facts, ma'am.

Researchers have discovered that chocolate produces
some of the same reactions in the brain
as marijuana.
The researchers also discovered other similarities
between the two but can't remember what they are.

Matt Lauer

Chapter 24

Good Mood Food

. . . .

Chocolate always puts me in a good mood, and many of us have turned to it for solace for a broken heart, in times of stress, or even a bad-hair day. I will actually use any excuse to get a bite of chocolate, but does it really enhance mood?

One study in San Diego, California, found that depressed people ate more chocolate. They did not draw the conclusion that eating chocolate causes depression, thank goodness, but rather that chocolate seems to elevate mood for approximately three minutes after eating. Perhaps the depressed folks were taking a moment to regroup and look on the sunny side of life? Not a bad strategy.

I am not terribly surprised to report that they also noted that when the chocolate was consumed without sugar or any sweetener to make it tasty, mood change was not present. Have you ever munched a spoonful of unsweetened cocoa or cooking chocolate? It is pretty nasty stuff.

On the other hand, eating chocolate stimulates the brain's production of endorphins, opioids that are also created by aerobic exercise. That's encouraging. Eating chocolate is associated with easing pain, soothing jangled nerves, hurt feelings, and big bummer days. All these good vibes come your way, not from the chemical reaction directly on the brain, but because we like eating chocolate and it gives us pleasure, so that part of the brain lights up.

In a study by Andrew Drewnowski, at the University of Michigan in 1995, binge eaters injected with an opiate receptor blocker ate less chocolate than before. Is this an indication of the opiate-like power of chocolate? Further studies are warranted and I would volunteer as a test subject. Are you in?

Dark chocolate also contains serotonin, the neurotransmitter your nerves produce. In addition to influencing your mood, serotonin also moves food through your intestines and helps constrict blood vessels. Dark chocolate with a cocoa level of over 85 percent may increase serotonin levels in the body from its fat and sugar content. Carbohydrates also signal the body to create more serotonin. The increase lasts only a couple of hours, but to my mind, that is enough to be a game or rather, mood changer.

Serotonin is made in the body, but is dependent on diet for tryptophan, an essential amino acid, for its creation. This amino acid is determined by what we eat. When fasting, serotonin levels drop.

Research by the Wellcome Trust and the Medical Research Council proved a connection between low serotonin levels and poor decision-making. Depression, obsessive-compulsive disorder (OCD), and aggressive behavior are also results of low serotonin levels. This explains why we are "not ourselves" when hungry, as one candy bar commercial shrewdly points out. It also points to an explanation for serotonin-rich foods like chicken soup and chocolate being considered comfort food.

Phenylethylamine (PEA) is found in high concentrations in the bodies of happy people. This neuromodulator enzyme is also found in high concentrations in dark chocolate and functions as a mood elevator and stimulant. Studies by Swiss researchers published in the *Journal of Proteome Research* in 2009 suggest that eating chocolate reduces stress hormones.

Another interesting ingredient in chocolate is the lipid, ananamide. This is chemically similar to tetrahydrocannabinol (THC), the active ingredient in marijuana, the one that makes you high. Activating the receptors for dopamine in the brain, ingestion of both substances cause people to feel great. In the brain, ananamide breaks down very quickly, but two other chemicals, which slow this breakdown, are also present in chocolate, extending the mood-enhancing effect.

You would have to eat twenty-five pounds of chocolate at a sitting to get the same high as from marijuana, but then you would also feel gross. Stick to the recommended one to two ounces a day and enjoy the heck out of it! Chocolate is, indeed a good mood food. It offers, through its pleasurable mouth feel, antioxidant content, and neuromodulators, a respite from the troubles of the day.

After eating chocolate you feel godlike, as though you can conquer enemies, lead armies, entice lovers.

Emily Luchetti

Chapter 25

Chocolate and Endurance

. . . .

I took a hike way back in my twenties and while this may not sound like a big deal, it was a very long hike and a pivotal experience for me. Regular workouts had not yet come into fashion in the early seventies, and if you were spotted running down the street, it was assumed someone was chasing you. I thought I was fit enough, being young, not overweight and all, but my hike from Washington State to California on the Pacific Crest Trail soon proved me wrong, so wrong.

My hiking partner and I headed out with a very short preparation period, subpar equipment, and one map of the Cascade Mountains. We hitchhiked (not recommended) across the country to the Columbia Gorge, where we camped for a few days before heading up, and I do mean up, the trail.

I had gotten the notion to join this acquaintance from having overheard that he was going on an epic hike and was looking for a companion. I set off with absolutely no idea what I was in for, endurance wise. Another friend had coached me on how to pack our food for optimum energy value. She was part of a mountain-climbing team, lucky for me, and gave me strict instructions on how to calculate calories needed throughout the day.

Making up little baggies of meals and snacks per her instructions, to ensure we would have the steam to make it up the trail, we sought calorie and protein-rich foods that would also be easy to cook. I am so grateful to that friend, for we encountered more than one hungry party on the trail who had miscalculated the sheer volume of food needed to complete the journey. We had enough to share with these unfortunates and, due to our careful preparations, we knew exactly how much we could spare.

Carrying my giant pack, I resented the necessity to haul all my nutrition every step of the way and quickly shed all nonessential items. One day we met a party of seasoned hikers headed north; they were hiking the entire Pacific Crest Trail from Mexico to Canada. We were impressed and even though it put our once proud goal of the whole span of Oregon a bit to shame, we admired them.

I admired them even more when they broke out large chunks of chocolate and began to chow down. They did not offer to share, but I didn't resent that, knowing how judiciously they must have calculated their caloric needs against the weight they were carrying. But I did envy them the chocolate! How can you carry that without having it melt all over your pack? I asked. Turns out it was a special hikers' chocolate with a higher melting point, which must have decreased its mouth feel, but still—chocolate!

A new study by scientists at the University of San Diego shows a definite connection between chocolate consumption and endurance. The study, which was done with mice, divided the group into two halves. One half was fed concentrated liquid polyphenols, such as you would get from eating chocolate, and the other half, water. Each half was divided again; one was set to a short daily walk on a treadmill, while the other half sat around looking pretty. After fifteen days, the mice were each given little endurance tests. Those that got the liquid polyphenols (the equivalent of a daily dose of dark chocolate) and walked a bit on a treadmill daily did 50 percent better than the control group.

Later when the mice were autopsied (which seems a poor reward for their contribution to science), it was found that the polyphenol-dosed mice had more mitochondria in their cells and and capillaries in their muscles than the mice who did not. More mitochondria indicate a healthier muscle that is less susceptible to fatigue. The mice that received the polyphenols but had no exercise did better than the non-polyphenol dosed mice, but by a much slimmer margin than those that had jogged on the treadmill.

The scientists concluded that while the exact mechanisms were not yet known, very small amounts of dark chocolate, such as half of one square or one-sixth of an ounce could intensify the effects of a workout.

Knowing this, I am inclined to hike the Pacific Coast Trail again, forty years later, to see if the addition of chocolate will make it easier for me. Truth is, that hike nearly killed me. I sprained both ankles in the first week, hated my pack with a ferocity I found difficult not to project on the guy who got me into this, and vigorously prayed for downhill stretches—that is, until I discovered the going down was almost as painful as the going up had been; it just shifted the pain to a different set of muscles.

If I ever go again, I will be sporting top-of-the-line equipment. My gear was simply not up to the rigors of the trip last time, and I arrived at the California border (oh, yeah, I made it) with almost every item leaking its stuffing, and a broken pack frame. But, boy was I in good shape!

Another thing—I will be packing daily doses of chocolate. One bit of good news about that study with the mice was that the amount of chocolate they were fed comes to about a half ounce per day in human terms—in other words, not enough to impact weight gain. I recommend at least an ounce to get the other benefits chocolate confers. Now, I just have to locate some freeze-dried wine and I'm all set for my next hike.

All you need is love, but a little chocolate
now and then doesn't hurt.

....

Charles M. Shultz

RADICAL INDULGENCE

Chapter 26

Love and Chocolate

· ·

They just seem to go together, don't they? Have the Valentines Day promoters of the traditional gift of chocolate sold us and our beloveds a bill of goods, or is there some basis in fact for the belief that chocolate is an aphrodisiac? Let me get this out of the way from the start. There is no scientific proof that eating chocolate improves sexual arousal or performance in men or women.

Don't tell Montezuma that (you can't, the Aztec leader has been dead for over eight hundred years). He reputedly consumed fifty goblets of the "food of the Gods" per day to keep up his strength and satisfy his six hundred wives. Well, Monte had more on his plate than your typical fella out to woo his girl, but still! This dramatic gesture seems to have launched a persistent rumor that chocolate is an aphrodisiac and many still swear by it, though there is no proof as of yet.

Chocolate does, however contain neurotransmitters (PEA and lipid anandamide) that activate dopamine reception and cause feelings of well being. Combined with the mild stimulant theobromine and the fact that it sensuously melts at body temperature, we might consider the combined effect an aphrodisiac.

As a proven mood enhancer, a gift of chocolate might be a good first move in the mating game. The sugar and carbohydrates in your gift could contribute to energy reserves that may be needed if you get lucky.

Chapter 27

Caffeine, Sleeplessness, and Chocolate

. . . .

A quick search on the web will net you a number of definitive answers to this question and those answers contradict themselves. Caffeine yes, caffeine no, what should you believe?

First, there is caffeine in the whole cocao bean; it is contained in small quantities in the hulls, which are discarded before processing into food products. Yes, there is actual caffeine in the chocolate after it is formed into bars or cocoa powder. The darker the chocolate, the more caffeine there is. Remember too, that the darker the chocolate, the less one typically eats! One pound of the darkest chocolate (90 percent cacoa) contains the caffeine of two cups of black tea. As one is unlikely to consume an entire pound (an ounce might be typical serving size) one can safely assume the effects of a sixth of a cup of black tea to be felt.

To be absolutely sure, avoid eating chocolate for three hours before bedtime. One bit of confusion seems to be that theobromine, the stimulant that is found in chocolate, is part of a family of methylxanthines that caffeine also belongs to. Theobromine is found in its most concentrated form in the cocao bean and has been shown to improve mood and blood pressure. It does have a stimulatory effect, but a much milder one than caffeine. It boosts blood sugar and also is a mild diuretic.

The way you feel after a good night's sleep is nothing short of a miracle, especially if you haven't had one in a while. Your mind is alert, and you are ready for the day in a whole new way after deep and restful sleep. Many people believe that chocolate disturbs their sleep and they avoid eating it after noon. As chocolate cravings often crop up late in the day, that is a lot of missed opportunity to indulge in the healthful practice of eating or drinking chocolate.

There is a bit of a mystery about the sleep-disturbing qualities of chocolate because it is a good source of tryptophan, the substance that launches serotonin production, which results in good sleep.

Still, sleeplessness might be caused by theobromine. Dark chocolate has more theobromine than those other forms, so you might want to avoid it a few hours before bedtime. The effect lasts only two to three hours, so you are cleared for your afternoon cup of hot chocolate, best made with soy, rice, or almond milk, as dairy blocks the absorption of the antioxidants in chocolate.

With its high PEA (phenylethylamine, another neurostimulant chemically similar to amphetamine) content, chocolate can elevate your mood, make you feel alert and excited, but might keep you awake, if you eat it right before bedtime. Nursing mothers are cautioned to avoid chocolate because of this effect, which can be exaggerated in the small bodies of their infants.

Theobromine acts differently in animals. Chocolate is a banned substance for racehorses because it acts as a stimulant in their systems. Dogs should never be given chocolate because of their inability to quickly process theobromine, which is poison to them.

Here is a fun fact: the longest living (documented) human was Jeanne Calment of France, who died in 1997 at the age of 122 years and 164 days. Among her dietary habits, which included ingesting olive oil and port daily, she ate a whopping two pounds of chocolate a week until she was 119. Not sure why she gave it up, but as she died soon thereafter, I guess one should stop eating chocolate at one's peril. Consider yourself warned.

Ms. Calment also rode a bike till she was one hundred years old and walked until she was one hundred and fifteen, when she broke her femur. Undoubtedly there was something special about her body and I do not recommend eating that much chocolate unless you have a similar constitution. Her chocolate consumption comes down to about 4.7 ounces of chocolate a day, which is three to four times the recommended daily amount—what a life!

What you see before you, my friend, is the result of a lifetime of chocolate.

....

Katherine Hepburn

Chapter 28

Chocolate Tips and Tricks

. . . .

Some people have a problem restraining themselves when chocolate is just lying around. Here are a few ideas to keep your habit in check. Coating a big crunchy rice cake with dark chocolate makes a satisfying snack—crunchy, generous, and oh so tasty.

Pull out the daily chocolate choice and leave the rest on a high shelf. Break it into small pieces and use as reward and enticement for yourself throughout the day. Eat the darkest chocolate you can tolerate. It has the highest antioxidant count and the sharp taste satisfies after a few bites. Don't eat your chocolate with dairy products as it is thought to block the absorption of the antioxidants in the gut. This means, (sorry) no milk chocolate.

To remember the recommended daily dose of your new healthy indulgences, follow the Three, Two, One Rule that I invented. Each day, have no more than:

- 3 cups of coffee
- 2 small glasses of red wine
- 1 ounce of dark chocolate

Wine

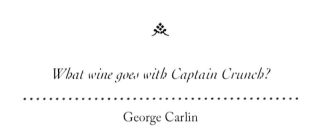

What wine goes with Captain Crunch?

George Carlin

Chapter 29

First Sips

. . . .

I have always enjoyed a good glass of wine and early on gradu-ated from light and fruity whites to dark and chewy reds—what I like to call "Load Bearing." Oh, I appreciate a good glass of white wine when appropriate—the steely Rieslings, oaky Chardonnays, crisp and bubbly Vinho Verde—but for me, they just go down too easily. I prefer to linger, to roll wine around in my mouth, to draw in a little air over the top of the taste to explode the flavor, and then swallow. I find it deliciously decadent, and every sip pleases and satisfies me.

Since my twenties, I have sipped a glass or two every evening as I prepare and enjoy dinner. Choosing and pouring is my signal that the work of the day is over and it's now time to shift into a different gear.

How wonderful to find that my daily red is not only a pleasure, but that it's good for me as well. There is a clue in the robust health of the Mediterranean population. In spite of their daily indulgence of a glass or two of tannic wine, copi-ous amounts of olive oil and butter, and regular indulgence in desserts, they enjoy longer lifespans than much of the world, Americans included. Enjoyment of food and drink is woven into the culture. In France, the quality of the wine, cheese, and bread is even regulated by law.

When one seeks value in every silky morsel and sip, how wonderful life can be! At age sixteen, I returned home from the school trip I took to Switzerland, ostensibly to study French, without having mastered the language, but madly in love with all things European. In the lovely town of Montreaux, in a fine old family hotel by Lake Geneva, I got my first taste of fabulously foreign food.

One evening we were taken to a local bistro where we ate creamy Swiss cheese like none I had ever tasted. Sliced so thin you could read through it, and paired with new wine served by handsome young men in lederhosen, this folksy evening designed for tourists seemed to punctuate our presence on foreign soil. With my first taste of wine—indeed alcohol in any form, save for a sip of Daddy's bourbon, which I thought tasted like ground-up toothpicks—I vowed to embrace a new level of sophistication in my life.

Our little group of young ladies and a few brave boys were astonished to be allowed to drink alcoholic beverages by our Swiss tour leaders. They must have been unfamiliar with the American custom of abstinence, especially for teenagers, for they encouraged us to enjoy ourselves and set no limit on our imbibing. So imbibe we did!

We stumbled and staggered home over steep cobbled streets to fall, bruised and happy, into bed. Next day found many of us missing the delicious breakfast rolls and cafe au lait, for we were too hungover to get out of bed. To say I felt rough for several days is an understatement. Forthwith, I would respect restraint and have been suspicious ever since of any drink that goes down too easily.

Switzerland is a land of mysterious rules and regulations. Woe to any visitor who inadvertently allows a slip of paper to fall from pocket or purse. Passersby will angrily chase you down and return the offending liter. We were strictly forbidden to chat with the Italian boys who hung around the lakefront, but it was apparently okay to buy a bottle of wine!

Encouraged by this loose attitude, and eager to push the limits while we could, some of us got together and bought a bottle of red wine, thinking it just might be easier on the system than that wonderful white we had tried the week before. I will always remember the label of that fine old St Emilion we drank by the water, hiding out of habit behind one of the statues that dotted the path around the lake.

I appreciated the castle on the bottle as I sipped the very strong, not very sweet wine from my little folding cup. I wanted to like it, but it was a lot to take, so many bold flavors and so different from any other beverage experience up till then. The best I could say at the time was that it was "good" (I did not want to be seen as unsophisticated), but maybe was an acquired taste.

My palate did not reject it outright and I thought perhaps I might recall the name of this wine to wow a date back home in the far distant future when I could legally order wine at a restaurant. At least I would know what to expect. It is now one of my favorites.

As we split the bottle among nine of us, no one got loaded and I vowed to give it another try, maybe when I was an adult. Turns out I had good instincts, because wine is not a recommended beverage for the bone-building years. Our bones grow and strengthen until our mid-to-late twenties, when they stop becoming stronger. After age forty or so, they weaken on their own every year. In my research, I discovered to my delight that a daily red wine habit can counteract this decline.

Chapter 30

A Brief History of Wine

. . . .

When the first housewife discovered that the grape juice went bad on the cave shelf, she must have said to herself, "Oh well, it's still grape juice, just a bit fizzy," and served it anyway. Not only was that evening around the cave fire an altogether more lively affair, but everyone got a good night's sleep for a change, untroubled by saber- tooth tiger roars or tummy upset, common, I would imagine, in a time before refrigeration. My imaginary cave wife probably began to stash some spare grape juice in the back of the cave cupboard for troubled times after the discovery that "bad" grape juice could be something very, very good.

One problem she and all successive generations, had up until bottles were invented, was that the goat stomach used to ferment and store wine lent it a decided pong. Indeed, for centuries people drank the wine, not for the mood elevating qualities or the taste—certainly not the taste—but because it made them sick less often than the water.

Paul Lukacs says in his book *Inventing Wine: A New History of One of the Worlds Most Ancient Pleasures* that the wine ancient people drank was "wretched, horrible, vinegary and foul." Its only redeeming quality was that the alcohol was a built-in disinfectant. This effect is borne out in a study by the University of Missouri-Columbia. They proved that red wine acts like an antimicrobial in the intestinal tract, countering food-borne pathogens.

In ancient Rome, they used wine as a water purifier of sorts. Drinking watered wine all day long might have had some unintended side effects. I'm thinking that the penchant for building aqueducts and creating indoor plumbing was born from a desire to make the side effects of excessive wine consumption more comfortable and convenient. It's a wonder they had the vim and vigor to conquer the world, half in the bag, as they were most of the time.

Wine, more than any other alcoholic beverage, has been a part of religious ceremonies. Wine was served at the Last Supper and in most churches the communion beverage is wine (not withstanding the Methodist practice of straight Welch's grape juice). Wine is part of the ritual on Passover. In his book *What would Jesus Drink?* Brad Whittington includes a list of all 247 verses in the Bible that refer to wine and strong drink, so you can easily read them for yourself and in context.

The modern era of winemaking began in the seventeenth century with the invention of the coal furnace, which made it possible to produce a sturdy glass wine bottle. Cleaner drinking water also became available about this time, so wine was not in demand as a water purifier. The quality of wine had to be stepped up to keep the market for wine strong. There had always been a broad range of quality in wines, and I am sure the patricians drank a much finer draft than the plebeians all through history.

With the advent of glass bottles to keep wine relatively uncontaminated, new wineries sprang up all over, in France especially. The winemakers built themselves chateaus in the ancient styles to create an image of a long history and the spin doctors began to weave their spell for wine drinkers worldwide.

The mysteries and mystique of winemaking began. The castle on the label of my first bottle of St. Emilion was not where winemaking began in this region of France, as I had imaginged. The the first wine was made there by Romans in the second century long before the medieval glories of princesses and knights who may have sampled this same claret.

Right now is the very best time to be a wine drinker. We have our choice of magnificently special (and expensive) wines and delicious, healthy vin ordinaire which is safe, affordable, and, best of all, delicious. To be sure, there are some very bad-tasting wines out there, but they are likely to taste bad to us because they are not to our taste rather than because they are truly and objectively foul.

Learning about wine is an engaging hobby that everyone can afford. You don't have to be a wine snob to enjoy wine daily. A fellow who came out to repair a leak in my camper water system confessed to being a "wino." Jim said he used to be a beer drinker, but now his passion is for wine. He travels around on his vacations visiting vineyards and sampling new wines, finding favorites from local and far-flung east coast locations. I applaud him for making an engaging hobby out of his own predilections. Jim was surprised when I told him that the wine he loved might be considered a health food!

Chapter 31

Wine Regions

. . . .

Wine is grown and produced in sixty-five countries of the world. Climate change is opening up new regions to production as fast as it is challenging others, so this is a dynamic statistic. There are over 6,000 vineyards producing wine in the US, and according to the Food and Agriculture Organization of the United Nations, the equivalent of 36 billion bottles of wine are produced worldwide each year.

Italy produces 17.53 percent of the world's wine, while France makes 16.17 percent and Spain produces 13.61 percent in an average for the years 2007-2010. The US follows at 10.56 percent. Good thing wine is good for you, because we seem to be drinking an awful lot of the stuff! How much? The Vatican City State tops the list for most wine per capita at 54.78 liters per year. That's per person! That was in 2010, down from 70.22 in 2009 (what in the world got into them that year?) That is an impressive amount of wine to guzzle.

The US comes in number one for per-capita consumption of the world's total wine production, followed by France and Italy. According to a 2010 list by the Wine Institute, there are 208 wine regions in the US in 31 states—who knew Oklahoma had wineries?

I was certainly surprised when I visited my home state of Virginia to discover some lovely wines being produced in over 200 vineyards located throughout six distinct regions in the state. Thomas Jefferson tried so hard to made a decent wine back in revolutionary times and apparently fell short. Whether from using modern tools and techniques or because of climate change, we now have a lot of delicious wine from unexpected sources right here at home in America.

I set out in "Little Bird," my trusty book tour van, with my dog Gracie (cheap date at the tasting rooms, as she is a teetotaler) to explore for myself this wonderful world of winemaking in America. My notes are available at the website for this book: www.RadicalIndulgence.com . There you will find a map of most wineries in the continental US and links to their web sites. I could not find a winery map that crosses state lines, so I made my own. It is most helpful when planning a trip or just wandering, to know where you might encounter the most delicious places for a break. This is an ongoing project and it is a good thing drinking wine adds to longevity, because it may take a while to personally get through the list.

What about organic wine? There are over two hundred pesticides commonly used on grapevines. They destroy not only pests, but the beneficial bacteria as well. Organic grow-ing practices retain flavor and the proper balance of natural sulfites for a delicious and healthful product. Think about it, wine from each wine region has it's own unique and wonderful qualities and by caring for the native soil and environment–the terroir–flavors are nurtured and enhanced. Find out more about organic wine at:www.organicvintners.com

*Quickly, bring me a beaker of wine, so that I may wet
my mind and say something clever.*

. . . .

Aristophanes

Chapter 32

Could Wine Really Be Good For You?

. . . .

The news is full of chirpy reports, such as "The latest research proves wine is great for your health, drink more wine!" While I rejoiced to hear the good tidings, I have a skeptical nature and went on the hunt to read the reports myself. I discovered a wealth of claims, studies, tests, surveys, and even more conclusions. Some gloomily admitted the limits of the study, others boldly proclaimed that a miracle of longevity and vigor was only a glass or two away.

Confused, I set out to sort it all for myself, and thus began my burning desire to share the facts, just the facts, ma'am. As you may have guessed, I have proved to my personal satisfaction that the consumption of wine—moderate consumption that is— offers positive benefits to health, as well as a spiritual, mental, and emotional boost that we can all take advantage of without feeling guilty.

Does drinking wine make you live longer? The old folks in France, Italy, and Greece seem to believe so. Researchers from the William Harvey Research Institute, Queen Mary's College, London, England, say that wine consumption is probably one of the contributing factors towards the long lifespans of Mediterranean peoples.

It is no accident that these people live longer; the wines of the area contain as much as ten times the amount of procyanidins as wine from other regions. Procyanidins (formerly called proanthocyanidins) are the most biologically active types of polyphenols. Higher concentration of procyanidins results from the long period of fermentation, three to four weeks, rather than the more modern method of one week.

The higher concentration of procyanidins makes the wine taste strongly of tannin. Consuming tannic wines yields an "overall sense of well-being and results in greater longevity," concluded Roger Corder, team leader of the research, who added, "There is a 19th century expression: A man is only as old as his arteries."

The Center for Alcohol Research in Copenhagen (there really is one, and it is not the clever name for a bar, but a real scientific outfit) has declared that, according to their new research, moderate drinking may help to extend lifespan. They found that a glass or two of wine or beer protects against heart disease, diabetes, and strokes, concluding that consistent moderate drinkers are more likely to outlive both heavy drinkers and teetotalers.

"The results show that alcohol can be good for your health, provided you adopt a careful drinking style," said Professor Morten Gronbaek, lead researcher. What he believes contributes to such happy outcomes is the lowering effect to LDL (bad cholesteral) along with the boost in HDL (good) cholesterol, which stops artery clogs.

✿

Not what we have, but what we enjoy, constitutes our abundance.

. . . .

Epicurus

Chapter 33

Lifespan

. . . .

Because the media so enthusiastically covered the discovery that resveratrol seemed to be linked to longevity in mice, I am devoting a section to address the claims and promise of resveratrol. The experiment that sparked a marketing resurgence for red wine as a miracle drug was done by Harvard Medical School professor of genetics David Sinclair.

In the study, one group of rats bred with genetic insulin resistance and obesity, (not a pretty group) were fed a diet containing 60 percent of their calories in the form of fat. The group was divided in two, and one half of the rats were fed resveratrol. Both groups continued to eat their high-fat diet. The rats receiving the resveratrol developed lower glucose levels. Their hearts and livers began to function better and they appeared to be more nimble on their tiny feet. They did not loose weight, but their health became as good as rats on a healthy diet while the nonresveratrol group sickened and died prematurely.

The resveratrol-fed rats lived a lifespan equal to the healthy rats. Note that it was not determined that lifespan was increased over that of the healthy rats. They only outlived the rats that were doomed to an early death by their lab-induced bad health.

"We think that aging is a component of many diseases or conditions, such as diabetes, Alzheimer's disease, and arthritis. Generally speaking, these occur later in life. The idea is that if you could target a molecule that could regulate the aging process, you could control these diseases." So says David Sinclair, Professor of Genetics at Harvard Medical School. Prof. Sinclair was a postdoc in Dr. Leonard Guarente's lab when the original research into the effects of resveratrol was done.

Scientists speculated that if the same effect could be duplicated in humans, then resveratrol could prevent the onset of type 2 diabetes, heart disease, and cancer in people predisposed to developing those health threats. In light of the epidemics of obesity and diabetes in the US now, this is mighty exciting stuff.

In addition to the dramatic physical effects on rats fed massive doses of resveratrol, scientists discovered an effect on a gene responsible for longevity—namely, SIRT1. The effect of resveratrol was postulated to be similar to that of caloric restriction on the so-called longevity gene, which seems to have the ability to extend life for many species, including the human variety. Resveratrol seemed to boost the cells' mitochondrial function in a way reminiscent of calorie restriction.

A restricted-calorie diet has been adopted by some as a way to extend life, a method that works well on yeast in a petri dish. To me, a life of constant hunger and less-than-satisfying meals would not be a life I would wish to last overlong. As a study of human lifespans takes, well, lifespans to conduct, the results have not been clear.

In recently concluded chimpanzee study, reduced-calorie diets proved ineffective at extending life. The Wall Street Journal reported that Rafael de Cabo, an experimental gerontologist at the US National Institute on Aging in Baltimore and lead author of the paper on the study, said, "One thing that's becoming clear is that calorie restriction is not a Holy Grail for extending the life span of everything that walks on earth."

A medication that could extend healthy years and life expectancy would be most welcomed by a society beset with rising medical costs and an ever-increasing aging population. Much debate has ensued over the efficacy of resveratrol in the years between the early trials and the present. Drug development was begun and abandoned, but new research seems to prove out the earlier claims.

Most recent is a study led by Clemens Steegborn at the University of Bayreuth in Germany, published in March 2013 in *Aging*. In his study, many of the earlier claims that resveratrol could indeed boost longevity seem to be vindicated.

The future of old age seems to be bright. "Ultimately, these drugs would treat one disease, but unlike drugs of today, they would prevent twenty others. In effect, they would slow aging. Now we are looking at whether there are benefits for those who are already healthy. Things there are also looking promising," says Sinclair, who now heads the Lowy Cancer Research Centre's Laboratory for Aging Research at UNSW. "We're finding that aging isn't the irreversible affliction that we thought it was" he says. "Some of us could live to age 150, but we won't get there without more research"

Some may bemoan the amount of money that changes hands in the pursuit of science, but somebody has to pay for all those PhDs to think through the results, and for all the experiments that don't pan out. The venture capitol that is put to use in this research not only advances science, but also yields unexpected bounty in the form of cures and preventions as yet undreamed of. I raise my glass in a toast to the men and women who dream and labor in the labs for the benefit of us all.

Chapter 34

What Should I Be Drinking?

· ·

If red wine is so good for you, how about other sources of alcohol, I wondered? You may have seen reports that beer and even spirits also have health benefits. Brace yourself, it's all true! So what should you drink? Choosing your poison can be easier when armed with a few facts. Here is a little crib sheet on the various benefits of different tipples.

The Hard Stuff

With spirits, the benefits from imbibing are mostly from the alcohol content. Sure, an amazing number of compounds come from plants and herbs and they might all have good effects of some kind. An excellent book on the topic, *The Drunken Botanist* by Amy Stewart contains a full rundown on the cornucopia of pharmacopeia that may be found in that special gin, cordial, or tipple of yours. Here are some of the good side effects of a good stiff drink:

- Lower blood pressure
- Better circulation
- Better cognition
- Reduced chance of Alzheimer's and dementia

A new study shows that three to five glasses of champagne a week can delay the onset of memory loss from dementia and Alzheimer's disease. Who wouldn't love that prescription?

Beer

By drinking beer one gets all the benefits of alcohol plus a healthy dose of minerals that contribute to heart health. There is such variety of beer, from Black Irish Ale to delicate rice beers from Japan, and all of them have something to recommend them—protein, B vitamins, phosphorus, magnesium, selenium, iron, niacin, and riboflavin, to name a few. To the beer lover, this is a bonus to the good side of alcohol. As Benjamin Franklin said, "Beer is living proof that God loves us and wants us to be happy."

White Wine

The benefits of white wine include all the benefits of alcohol but lack the added bonus of polyphenols which boost anti-inflammatory effects and contribute too the ability to build bone in later life. There is some research into developing a white wine with a greater antioxidant punch, but for now, it's the alcohol that is the main benefit of white wine.

Red Wine

Red wine has the Powerball Jackpot of health benefits, including all of the above effects plus the ability to lower glucose in the body, giving red-wine drinkers the edge in fat burning and lean-muscle building. The biggest bonus to red wine is the antioxidant advantage. Tannins and polyphenols including resveratrol it contains contribute mightily to one's health.

While a relatively small dose of resveratrol found in a glass or two of red wine has been recently found to have a more effective result than was originally supposed, there are other antioxidants in red wine that can lower the incidence of heart disease, build stronger bones, aid in circulation, and a create a sharper brain.

Some vintnors are working to increase the anti-oxident content of their wines. Owner and winemaker Amy LaBelle of LaBelle Winery in Amherst, New Hampshire wanted to let wine drinkers know that her wine with blueberries as an ingredient was high in anti-oxidents, but regulations do not allow such valuable information to be placed on wine labels.

What if I don't want to drink alcohol?

Red grape juice contains polyphenols as does nonalcoholic red wine and you can expect similar benefits from drinking it. You do lose out on the boost to circulation of alcohol, as well as the tannins and other flavonoids present in red wine, but this is a great choice if drinking does not work for you. Blueberry juice and pomegranate juice are also good. These may be found in juice concentrate without sugar for a more health-conscious mixer with sparkling water.

I make a mean sangria from non-alcoholic red wine with blueberry and cranberry concentrate, plus citrus from fresh limes and oranges. Ice down a pitcher of this and add a splash of non-alcoholic champagne for an excellent NA cocktail option.

Be sure your low-test wine has been de-alcoholized *after* fermenting, for the alcohol helps dissolve the antioxidants, making it a richer source than plain grape juice. It will be labeled as non-alcoholic wine rather than sparkling grape or apple juice.

Chapter 35

For a Healthy Heart - Have a Drink!

· ·

The older you are, the more careful you must be about your alcohol consumption. That does not sound like a recipe for fun—but wait. To maintain a healthy heart, research has shown that regular, moderate drinking has a proven benefit. So, take care to have that glass of wine or cocktail daily. Convivial cheer and a long healthy life; what could be better?

Light to moderate alcohol consumption has been shown to lower the risk of cardiovascular disease among the elderly. To get this particular benefit, one does not have to limit the fun to wine; any spirited liquid will do. Wine contains from 12 to15 percent of alcohol by volume. A glass of wine, (5 ounces) is the equivalent of a shot, 1.6 ounces of spirits, or 12 ounces of beer.

A study was conducted by the Institute on Aging in Gainesville Florida, tracking 2,500 people aged seventy to seventy-nine, none of whom showed evidence of heart disease when the study began. Half of the test subjects were light to moderate drinkers, and half had never touched a drop of alcohol. Over a period of five-and-a-half years, 307 died and 383 suffered a cardiac event. Those who drank up to seven alcoholic drinks a week were 27.4 percent less likely to die than those who abstained completely, and those same tipplers were 29 percent less likely to suffer a cardiac event.

While the team, led by Dr. Cinzia Maraldi, was not sure why moderate drinking helped, they speculated the benefit may be at the cellular level or caused by genetic factors, which interact with alcohol. Whatever the reason, this study is a sign that modest imbibing can not only improve the quality of life, but also extend it. Remember, this recommendation is for moderate drinking. If you overindulge, the benefit is lost and so is your good health.

High Blood Pressure

Hypertension (high blood pressure) can cause fibrosis, a hardening or stiffening of the heart tissue. Overactive cardiac fibroblasts secrete excess collagen that, in normal amounts, provides structure to heart tissue. The excess collagen prevents efficient pumping action, the heart's basic function.

At the Northeastern Ohio Universities Colleges of Medicine and Pharmacy (now Northeast Ohio Medical University), Associate Professor J. Gary Meszaros led a study on how the body tries to repair a damaged heart. The team of research scientists found that the body attempts to repair the heart by producing the angiotensin hormone at a high level to increase blood pressure. This plan backfires badly; the effect of the hormone causes cardiac fibroblast production to go into overdrive, creating a stiffening of the heart muscle. This, in turn, forces the heart to work harder to pump the blood supply around the body, and so further damages the organ.

This study was done with rats that had the condition of cardiofibrosis. When the scientists pretreated the rats' cardiac fibroblasts with resveratrol, the effect was to inhibit the large quantities of collagen usually produced when the angiotensin was present, as is the case when hypertension leads to overactive fibroblasts.

They concluded, and the American Heart Association agreed, that one or two glasses of red wine a day could reduce the damage that runaway collagen production does to a heart. They noted that the amount of resveratrol in a glass of wine varies according to variety, but agreed that nearly all types of dark red varieties—merlot, cabernet, zinfandel, shiraz, and pinot noir—had enough to be of help.

French researchers reported in the *FASEB Journal*, published by the Federation of American Societies for Experimental Biology, that polyphenols, found in abundance in wine and chocolate and coffee, facilitate the growth of blood vessels and thus promote better circulation. They found that adding one glass of red wine per day could create a measurable effect. Brightly colored fruits and vegetables and juices also contain polyphenols.

"When it comes to finding treatments for complex diseases, the answers are sometimes right there waiting to be discovered in unexpected places like the produce aisles or wine racks of the nearest store," said Gerald Weissmann, MD, and editor-in-chief of the *FASEB Journal.* He went on to say, "But it takes modern science to isolate the pure compound, test it in the lab, and and go on from there to find new agents to fight disease."

His statement brings me back to a point I made earlier in this book: all of these substances have broad appeal. True, not everyone craves all three—coffee, chocolate, and wine (I am one of the lucky ones who love that kind of medicine)—but isn't it interesting that we humans gravitate towards what is good for us, then deny ourselves those very substances in a false belief that, in denial, we are doing what is good and healthful.

I believe that if I ingest the food and drink that are right for my body, I can establish a truce of sorts with my cravings. When I am well nourished by food I love, then I can enjoy all I want of the treats that should be enjoyed in moderation, trusting that I will "want" just the right amount.

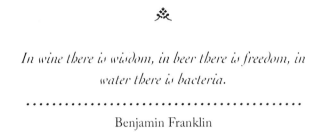

In wine there is wisdom, in beer there is freedom, in water there is bacteria.

....

Benjamin Franklin

Chapter 36

Alcohol and Cancer

. . . .

We hear a lot about the apparent controversy between the drinkers and nondrinkers regarding cancer. Is it good or is it bad? The answer, as with so many tricky questions, is an equally tricky "It depends . . ." Some researchers say wine causes more cancer than it cures or prevents, and the American Cancer Institute says it is a good tool for cancer prevention, a tennis tournament of opinions.

Alcohol can raise hormone levels in women, which has been connected to higher incidence of breast cancer. If you are at risk for breast cancer, it would seem best to avoid drinking. There are genes that indicate risk, so if you really want to know, get tested.

This testing cannot be undertaken lightly; counseling and a full family history are required, because the options if the gene mutation is present—the BRCA1 or BRCA2 gene—can be extreme. Knowing your risk can help you and your family make important healthcare decisions and may help you decide if a drink a day is a good idea for you.

How it works
Red wine is a good source of polyphenols, such as catechins and resveratrol, which are thought to have antioxidant or anti-cancer properties. Resveratrol is an antioxidant and a type of polyphenol called a phytoalexin, which is produced as part of a plant's defense system against disease, such as invading fungus,

stress, injury, infection, or ultraviolet irradiation. Red wine contains high levels of resveratrol, as do grapes, raspberries, peanuts, and other plants.

Polyphenols are antioxidant compounds found in the skin and seeds of grapes. When wine is made from these grapes, the alcohol produced by the fermentation process dissolves the polyphenols contained in the skin and seeds. Red wine contains more polyphenols than white wine because the making of white wine requires the removal of the skins after the grapes are crushed. The phenols in red wine are thought to be responsible for holding the line against oxygen damage—antioxidants.

We need oxygen to live, but under certain situations, it has deleterious effects on the human body. Most of the potentially harmful effects of oxygen are due to the formation and activity of a number of chemical compounds. These compounds are the building blocks of free radicals, molecules that can damage the membranes of cells by attacking the important molecules of proteins, carbohydrates, lipids, and DNA.

Cellular damage caused by free radicals has been implicated in the development of cancer and in problems of aging in general. Antioxidants protect cells from oxidative damage caused by free radicals.

Research on the antioxidants found in red wine has shown that they may help inhibit the development of certain cancers. Research at the Bordeaux University in France concluded that a glass of wine a day could keep blood circulation brisk and prevent clogs. This study also found that high doses of polyphenols shut down and prevent cancerous tumors by cutting off formation of new blood vessels needed for tumor growth.

The dose to achieve this effect was high, the equivalent of a full bottle of red wine per day. This is obviously too much wine to be healthy, but they postulated that the polyphenols could be extracted and given in higher doses as needed without that tipsy feeling. Remember too, the other sources of resveratrol such as grapes, raspberries, and other red-skinned fruit can be included in one's daily diet to round out a full dose per day.

There is growing evidence that the health benefits of red wine are related to its non-alcoholic components. Nonalcoholic red wine has the same properties as the high-test beverage, as long as the alcohol was removed after creating the wine. Remember that the polyphenols use the alcohol to dissolve their potent qualities into the wine.

The final word on using resveratrol for treating disease is not yet in. This is complex topography and there are many teams of scientists on the case, diligently working with their computer models and gene splicers to effect cures. You don't have to rush out and buy resveratrol tablets; you don't really know what's in them, nor is the proper dose sorted out just yet. I'd stick to a glass or two of a favorite red wine or a pitcher of non-alcoholic sangria, and wait for news from the biotechies.

More Proof

Here are the results of a few more studies on red wine (and the polyphenols it contains) as a cancer-preventative agent. Resveratrol has been shown to reduce tumor incidence in animals by affecting one or more stages of cancer development. It has been shown to inhibit growth of many types of cancer cells in culture by reducing the activation of NF kappa B, a protein produced by the body's immune system when it is under attack. This protein affects cancer-cell growth.

The cell and animal studies of red wine have looked into effects on several cancers, including leukemia, skin, breast, and prostate cancers. Evidence from animal studies suggests this anti-inflammatory compound may be an effective chemo-preventive agent in three stages of the cancer process: initiation, promotion, and progression.

Research studies published in the *International Journal of Cancer* show that drinking a glass of red wine a day may cut a man's risk of prostate cancer in half and that the protective effect appears to be strongest against the most aggressive forms of the disease. It was also seen that men who consumed four or more four-ounce glasses of red wine per week have a 60 percent lower incidence of the more aggressive types of prostate cancer.

Cancer Risks

The story is different for women. Because alcohol raises estrogen levels, there is an increased risk of breast cancer among even moderate female drinkers. Reviewing your family and health history, taking into account any hormone therapies and steroid use, can help you decide whether to take that risk for the other benefits of moderate drinking.

There are increased levels of other types of cancer as well, including mouth, throat, esophagus, liver, and rectum. Taking a look at your overall health picture will be a help in determining your safe if any level of alcohol intake. Armed with the facts, you are ready to make wise, healthful, and delicious choices for yourself. À votre santé!

Beer is made by men, wine by God.

Martin Luther

Chapter 37

Alcohol and Brain Health

. . . .

Here is some good news for people who value their thought processes and hope to avoid dementia as they age. Moderate red wine drinkers develop dementia less often than abstainers. A study by the Australian National University, drawing results from ten scientifically rigorous research projects involving more than 10,000 people worldwide, found that moderate drinkers were 28 percent less likely to develop Alzheimer's disease than nondrinkers. Twenty-five percent were less likely to develop vascular dementia, and 26 percent were less likely to develop any type of dementia. I like those odds.

The evidence proved true for men and women alike and there was no differentiation between various types of alcohol. Professor Kaarin Ansley, who heads the Aging Research Unit at the Centre for Mental Health Research, Australian National University, Canberra, was not certain what caused the effect, but postulates that the protective effects of alcohol consumption on reducing inflammation and the benefits of socialization may be factors.

Researchers have recently been exploring the relationship of resveratrol (an active polyphenol in red wine) to cancer growth and brain disorders like Alzheimer's and dementia. They found that resveratrol aided in the formation of new nerve cells, which might make it useful in the treatment of Parkinson's and Alzheimer's.

Please remember that the good effects of alcohol on brain health are completely reversed by excessive consumption. Recent research shows that up to 20 percent of those diagnosed with Alzheimer's and dementia do not have those conditions. Their symptoms are, instead, a result of an alcoholic lifestyle. Binge drinkers seem especially susceptible to brain difficulties in later life. Binging even once a month increases risk, not only for dementia and Alzheimer's. For women, binge drinking of four to five drinks increases the risk of breast cancer by 55 percent. Heavy alcohol use and binge drinking can also increase the risk of pancreatic cancer in men.

The Royal College of Psychiatrists in the UK says people over sixty-five should drink a maximum of only 1.5 units of alcohol a day, the equivalent of one small glass of wine or a half-pint of beer. Their research postulates that older people do not process alcohol as quickly or as well as younger people. They worry that the older problem drinkers are being ignored by their physicians, and that there may be prescription drug complications with alcohol consumption.

Emma Soames, editor of *Saga Magazine*, says of this report, "I think people will be infuriated by this. It's described as a public health problem; it's actually a private health matter." She worries that the caution will be entirely discounted by the "ridiculously low" recommended daily allowances.

In the US one drink per day is the recommended limit for women, while two drinks a day are the allowance for a man. See the chapter "Choose Your Poison" for more details on measurements, alcohol content, and dose.

If you are wondering if you have slipped at all as you age, there is a test to compare your performance to your peers. It is called the MMSE—Mini Mental State Exam. A contradiction to the recent UK study on the damage alcohol can do to memory, women who had up to two drinks a day scored 20 percent higher than abstainers or occasional drinkers. This study, done at College of Physicians and Surgeons of Columbia University in New York, covered 3,298 residents of northern Manhattan and was adjusted for risk factors such as income, marital status, race, and ethnicity.

The fact is, each body and age are different. Pay attention to your overall health. There may be times when less alcohol is better. Just because I am making a case for indulgence does not mean I am advocating pulling out all the stops. Because alcohol reduces the ability to make good judgment, it would be wise to err on the side of caution in how much you drink. Setting limits before you imbibe definitely makes sense.

Either give me more wine or leave me alone.

Rumi

Chapter 38

Wine and Bone Health

. . . .

One of the most thrilling and surprising facts I unearthed in my research is the news that drinking red wine contributes significantly to bone health. Loss of strong bones is a concern as we age, and rightly so. It is hard to regain one's mobility and agility after a fall in old age. One in two postmenopausal women and one in four men will break a bone due to bone loss in their lifetime, according to the US National Institutes of Health.

Osteoporosis is the name of this thinning bone condition and it means, quite literally, "porous bone." Bones are not a solid mass of matter but a honeycomb-like collection of protein, calcium, and other minerals that make up the struts of bone. Beneath a solid outer layer, the mesh of the inner bone looks to be about two-thirds solid tissue and one-third spaces. In a bone suffering from osteoporosis, the struts become long and thin and the spaces are enlarged. This makes for a much more brittle bone.

Women and men alike form and lose bone every day. We are constantly in the process of remaking bone. Bits of bone dissolve and are carried away while a deposit of new bone cells is laid down. The cells whose job it is to break down bone are called osteoclasts while the cells responsible for building bone are called osteoblasts.

The osteoclasts are industrious little critters and they do not hesitate when they believe there is work to be done. Say you break your arm and it languishes in a cast for two months.

Without the muscle pulling on the bone via the tendons and ligaments, the bone has really no purpose. Bone is taken away when it is no longer in use. The osteoclasts get busy and in no time at all your now mended arm is a shadow of its former self in thickness and density. You must do some kind of physical of therapy—lift a weight or scrub a muffin tin to call that bone back into service. Stressing that weak bone will get the osteoblasts busy laying down new bone.

The biggest risk factor for osteoporosis is heredity. Seventy to eighty percent of bone strength is genetically determined. Do some checking to find out the state of your parents' and grandparents' bones. Frequent fractures in their later life could mean you are more likely to face thinning bones yourself.

Where does drinking red wine come in? A twin study in England showed startling results. In the study, 1,000 pairs of twins in their midfifties were the test subjects. Twins are a perfect group to compare because the genetic makeup is so similar it reduces the variations due to environment and genetics. It was discovered that when half the women drank a glass or two of red wine daily, their bone density was 20 percent greater than that of their sister abstainers.

Lead researcher Urszula Iwaniec at Oregon State University's Skeletal Biology Laboratory discovered the key players in the rebuilding of bones in the wine-drinking women. She proved that moderate consumption of red wine got the osteoblasts all riled up and ready to build bone. After two weeks of abstinence the evidence was clear that bone was being resorbed (taken away) in the forty postmenopausal female test subjects. Less than a day after resuming drinking, the markers of bone turnover returned to their previous levels in the wine-drinking half of test subjects. Bone building was back in progress! It appears that wine acts like estrogen to slow the loss of bone.

It is important to remember that while a drink or two a day can improve bone health, more than that tips the balance towards bone loss. Binge drinking is even more detrimental. Get clinical as you imbibe and keep in mind that the right dose size is vital to ensure the results.

I got out a measuring cup and carefully chose the size of my wine glass, making it easier for me to remember the right amount for my daily bone-strengthening draft. Then I picked a smaller glass so the wine amount looked satisfyingly generous!

What about other alcoholic beverages? Is wine the only pleasure that contributes to healthy bones? Dr. Katherine Tucker of Tufts University agrees that keeping track of the health benefits of alcohol is tough these days. "It is very confusing for people because alcohol has such diverse effects on different things," she said. Nevertheless, the effect of alcohol on bone mineral density (BMD) that she and the other researchers saw is "larger than we see from any other single nutrient, even calcium. It's not ambiguous. It's very clear."

Her study was made up of 1,182 men and 1,289 postmenopausal women, plus 248 premenopausal women all ranging in age from twenty eight to eighty-six. Men who had a glass or two of beer or wine a day had denser bones than abstainers, but the men who drank more than two shots of hard alcohol had lower BMD than the nondrinkers. Unfortunately, there was not enough data from the women to compare the effect of beer and wine on bone density because most of the women in the study preferred wine.

Tucker postulated that the alcohol might help build bones by boosting estrogen levels, which also accounts for increased breast cancer risk for women drinkers. It is never too late to build stronger bones and there is much that can be done without resorting to medical intervention.

If you believe you are at risk for osteoporosis, tell your doctor and point out your family history. The test to see how your bones are faring as you age is a scan called a Duel Energy X-ray Absorptiometry scan (DEXA scan). This is a noninvasive procedure and uses low doses of radiation. It takes only ten minutes to measure the bone density of lower spine and hips, which is an indictor of general bone health.

The medical remedies for bone loss can be inconvenient to take and can have unpleasant side effects, so prove to be ineffective in regaining youthful bone strength, as they are often not taken as prescribed. (Note that I am not recommending you drop your medication.) You might want to try these good health practices for a few months and notice how your bones are doing at your next scan.

•Keep bone strong by including calcium-rich foods in the diet.
• Get adequate sunshine for intake of vitamin D, needed to absorb the calcium.
• Do load-bearing exercise-lifting weights
• Drink a glass of red wine each day

The Framingham Heart study showed stronger bones in postmenopausal women who were moderate drinkers. Why all the focus on women and bone strength? Women generally have no trouble keeping their bones firm and strong throughout their reproductive years. After menopause, the rate of reabsorption (bone loss) increases due to less estrogen in the system, and the formation of new bone does not keep up with the loss. The net result is an overall loss of bone density.

The good news is that you can stimulate bone growth any time you want—provided you are not waiting around for a break to mend—by starting a weight-training program. That is a fast way to rebuild porous bones and anyone can do it.

Here is how weight training builds bone. Bone that is not stressed is neatly broken down by the osteoclast cells and carted off to be reabsorbed into the body. Bone that is stressed has a reason to be there and the osteoclasts get to work at that site to lay down new bone. When a muscle contracts, it pulls on the bone via the ligament, thus stressing the bone.

The best way is to lift as heavy a weight as you can manage for ten reps or as many as you can do. This stresses the bone so that it builds itself up. Then wait a week for the next go-around. This takes about twenty minutes a week once your routine is set, so no excuses—just do it. Don't worry; you won't get massive muscles bulging out from under your t-shirt, but you just may loose an inch or two by reshaping the muscle.

Get the advice of a professional on your weight-lifting form so you don't injure yourself as you begin. Don't overdo it! The rewards become setbacks if you pull a muscle and have to lay off the weights for a month or two.

Here is some good news for the heavyset. Just hauling your extra pounds around works to keep your bones strong. Of course you have to go out there and actually move about to make this work. Stair climbing and mountain walks are easy ways to add to bone density for people of all sizes.

Note that being of slight build puts one at greater risk for osteoporosis and extra weight bearing exercise is needed to compensate. I like the one-to-three pound hand weights. These can strap to your wrists or be held as you walk to double up the effects of your exercise time.

An added benefit is that lifting weights makes metabolism more efficient. Eat a high-protein, low-carb diet to support your strength training, and you will be rewarded by a strong body that grows more shapely as time goes by. When your muscles have a reason to live, just like your bones, because they called into action on a regular basis, they reward you by burning calories more efficiently.

That's right; with a higher metabolic rate you can justify all those extra calories from all the chocolate and wine I am recommending you add to your diet. Being slim, strong, and happy to be alive that much longer is a great side effect of all your thoughtful indulgence.

As lifespans get longer, it is vital that we take every precaution to also increase our youth span. No one wants to be a frail old thing. It is possible to retain vigor and bone density through all the stages of life. It is never too late to build and protect bones. I'll propose a toast to our continued bone health, right after my mountain walk.

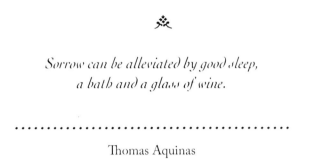

Sorrow can be alleviated by good sleep,
a bath and a glass of wine.

. . . .

Thomas Aquinas

Chapter 39

Choose your Poison

. . . .

Now that you are armed with the facts and have decided to become a dedicated moderate drinker, how do you decide what and how much you should drink? You may be wondering, with all the caution about moderation, exactly what constitutes the right dose for you? That depends on what effect you want. If you are looking to build bone, stick to red wine. If you just want to add to your brain health, drink whatever you like, but stick to the proper dose.

How much alcohol is there in a drink? The Center for Disease Control was my source for the following information:

A standard drink is 14.0 grams or 0.6 ounces of pure alcohol. This amount of alcohol equaling one drink is found in:

- 12 ounces of beer.
- 8 ounces of malt liquor.
- 5 ounces of wine.
- 1.5 ounces or a "shot" of 80 proof distilled spirits or liquor (rum, vodka, or my personal favorite, scotch).

International guidelines for daily consumption vary greatly, from a low of five drinks a week for a woman and ten for a man in Poland, to a high of twenty-one for women and twenty-eight for a man in the United Kingdom. Italy, Spain, and France recommend identical limits for men and women alike.

In the United States, the Department of Agriculture, Department of Health and Human Services, National Institute of Alcohol Abuse and Alcoholism, and the American Heart Association all recommend that men consume no more than fourteen drinks a week, and that women limit themselves to seven drinks a week. I personally believe it should relate to body weight. If you like precision, here is a handy method to calculate your optimum daily wine intake precisely.

According to the Center for Disease Control, the average weight of an American male over age twenty equals 195 pounds. The average weight of an American female over age twenty is 166 pounds.

If a man at 195 pounds can metabolize the alcohol in two drinks safely, then a woman should be able to safely imbibe and metabolize 1.70 drinks per day. If wine is your drink, with the usual pour of five ounces, a man can drink ten ounces and a woman eight and a half ounces, or a little over a glass and a half. Make adjustments according to your actual weight.

Problem Drinking

While I am advocating the extreme enjoyment of a glass of wine or two, I am aware that drinking poses a big problem for some people. My own father used alcohol to ease the pain of his chronic arthritis and became addicted.

As Dad readily admitted, he loved to drink, but he was eventually able to see that it did not serve him, his life purpose, or our family, to carry on with his favorite pain management practice. He quit cold turkey and promptly fell apart physically. It seemed the alcohol was the only thing keeping his body together. Alcohol is, in fact the only addictive substance that is able to kill you if you stop using it abruptly.

Tragically, some people cannot overcome the compulsion to drink, no matter how great their desire and motivation to do so. Alcoholism or alcohol dependence is defined by the American Medical Association (AMA) as "a primary, chronic disease with genetic, psychosocial, and environmental factors influencing its development and manifestations."

Because of the family history of alcoholism, I have kept a close eye on my own drinking. Having a low tolerance for alcohol was a positive sign. I just can't drink much. To enjoy getting drunk, I must pay close attention, as the fun never lasts long. I usually fall asleep after two drinks. As a drinker, I'm not exactly the life of the party, and the three-day hangover I get every time I overdo it is enough to discourage me from excess.

Non-alcoholic Wine

Many people who don't choose to drink wine are sick and tired of hearing all about how they ought to. What about non-alcoholic wine? Does it offer the same benefits as the loaded stuff? Sometimes I want to drink more than I should and use the "decaf" version (no, there is no caffeine in wine, just my bad joke about wine sans the alcohol). Mixing it with the good stuff seems a terrible waste, so I use it to make an antioxidant rich beverage that tastes like sangria without the headache.

Here is my recipe:
- One bottle non-alcoholic red wine
- 1/2 orange, thinly sliced
- 1/2 lemon or lime, thinly sliced
- 1 T Truvia or equivalent sugar or non-calorie sweetener
- 1/2 c pitted red cherries, or berries, if desired

Mash the citrus with muller or back of a spoon in a big pitcher, stir in other ingredients and chill. Add a splash of non-alcoholic champagne or soda water if desired and garnish with the fruit.

Does non-alcoholic wine or beer contain any alcohol? Nonalcoholic wine generally contains about one percent alcohol and orange juice a mere 0.2 to 0.4 percent. Nonalcoholic beer contains 0.4 percent alcohol. In the US and many other countries, any drink with less than 0.5 percent alcohol can legally be described as non-alcoholic, because your body can metabolize the alcohol as fast as you consume the drink. Although all orange juice contains alcohol, the quantity is low enough that you won't get intoxicated from it, even if you drink many glasses. However, in places with zero-tolerance rules against driving with any measurable alcohol in your blood, you might need to be careful if you are a very heavy orange juice drinker!

Does non-alcoholic wine deliver the goods?A new study reported in an online journal–*Circulation Research*, Spanish researchers found that of sixty-seven men with high cardiovascular or diabetes risk factors, there was a drop in blood pressure when drinking two glasses of non-alcoholic wine per day. The drop was modest, but was enough to significantly reduce their risk of coronary incidents and stroke. The men were also tested while drinking gin and regular red wine.

The polyphenols in the red wine, it seems, persisted through the de-alcoholization process. Keep in mind that the polyphenols dissolve in the alcohol, so be sure to use the non-alcoholic wine rather than grape juice. Grapes are also high in polyphenols but they are less available in that form.

There were a few problems with this study, due to the small group of test subjects and the fact that they knew what was being ingested—seriously, who wouldn't be able to tell red wine from gin? There was an insignificant "washout" period between each session with a particular drink, so some of the benefit might actually be a carryover from the previous test.

The good news here is that non-alcoholic red wine contains the same amount of polyphenols as the regular stuff and may be consumed expecting the same or even greater health benefit.

Chapter 40

Drinking Tips and Tricks

. . . .

When it comes to drinking, it is all too easy to overdo it. If alcohol has become a problem in your life, don't mess around, get help right away. Some people are more susceptible to the effects of alcohol, and when it drives the bus, instead of you—well, the passenger of that bus is at the mercy of an impaired person.

Remember the recommended maximum alcohol consumption for a woman is between one to two drinks per day; for men, up to three. These are small glasses, five ounce glasses, not full-to-the-brim balloon glasses. Measure your shot and see how it looks in different glasses so you can be a good judge without geekily pulling out your jigger measure at the table. See the section "Choose Your Poison" for guidelines.

That said, a glass of wine could be one of the most enjoyable rituals of your day. Make sure to cultivate a taste for red wines. In order to savor it, do a bit of prep work. As any alcoholic beverage can dehydrate as well as elevate, be sure you have kept up with your body's needs for liquid before imbibing. During the warm months, at higher altitudes, and when doing a lot of walking, the need for moisture can be hard to keep up with. Older people should pay special attention because they become dehydrated faster than the young.

A tall glass of iced tea (I use decaf or herbal, as even the small amount of caffeine keeps me up if I drink it in the afternoon) is a good start while waiting for or preparing dinner. To stall the beginning of what I like to call "Wine o'Clock," I have a sweet. One square of dark chocolate elevates the mood and staves off the desire for a glass of wine. I find that if I can put off quaffing until I have prepared dinner and sit down to eat, my five to eight ounce daily allotment is a lot more satisfying. Sometimes I go wild and have a thimbleful more for dessert.

When you begin your cocktail hour at a certain time each day, your body begins to expect a hit of sugar about that time every day. It gets upset with you for denying this expected treat and makes you feel dissatisfied. A cup of sugar-free hot chocolate or cool lemonade sweetened with Truvia between four and five o'clock each day will be a satisfying way to hold off until you are fully ready to enjoy and savor your wine.

My dad used to eat a couple of cookies or a piece of cake to get him past his evening Jim Beam craving after he gave up the drink. It worked well for him, but he had to adjust his diet accordingly. The saying "Eat dessert first; life is uncertain" could really work for you here.

When you are ready for your glass of wine, make it a special one. Note I did not say expensive. There are many fine and interesting wines to be had for under ten dollars. Another big advantage of reining in your drink consumption is that you can afford a splurge now and again because you go through fewer bottles.

When I travel, I consult my map of wineries (you can find it on the book website: www.RadicalIndulgence.com) and make time to drop in on a new tasting room along the way. I get a nice break, tasting and choosing my new favorites and chatting with the vintner. When I find something really special, I buy a case on the spot. Master the art of spitting out your taste and you will be able to drive on to your business without impairment, or else go late in the day with a friend and make an evening of it.

Just be sure someone is abstaining so you both get home safely.

Drink a glass or two of water for each glass of wine. This will keep your teeth white, your body hydrated, and ensure that when you do take a sip, your palate will be clear.

Chapter 41

To Sum It All Up

· ·

Always eat and drink the very best coffee, chocolate, and wine you can find and afford. Branch out and try variations of your favorites to enhance your pleasure. Appreciate every sip and morsel. Note how your body reacts and makes use of your treat, and learn how to use each wisely to enrich your life. A bite of chocolate in the afternoon to sharpen the mind, a strong espresso after a big meal to keep you energized for the theater, the comfort of a glass of wine after a long day—these are riches that anyone can afford.

Taking the time to honor your own needs by enjoying a break, then returning to your work refreshed, is surely worth the sacrifice of a few productive moments in the workday. Relax Puritan restraint and sink into the world of indulgence, armed with the understanding that it is all so very good for you.

Use the results of the studies in this book to your own advantage and tailor your dose of indulgence accordingly. Sometimes the medicine goes down pretty darn easily, even without a spoonful of sugar.

Acknowledgements

To my parents and grandparents, (and especially my mother, who is an amazing cook,) thank you for showing me how to savor life's pleasures, small and large, to prize the rare, to appreciate the excellent and to save a piece for my brother, however difficult that is.

I offer gratitude to Jenny Garden, my editor who labored over the smallest piece of punctiation and politely told me "No." (I could not use the phrase "a bit" twenty-four times in one small book.)

Many thanks for the friendship, creative spirit and talent of Carolina Palermo Schulze, creator of the amazing cover photograph-*La Bacchante with homage to Caravaggio.*

For Tracey Bowman, friend and previous co-author who delivered a constant stream of encouragement and friendship as well as a great critical eye, I am always grateful.

Appreciation goes out to Spencer Zahn, who advised, cajoled, and tactfully proded me to do a better job on the front and back covers.

Thanks to FancyHands, my research partners who ferreted out the facts, studies, opinions and claims that formed the foundation of the book.

Finally, I appreciate Gracie, my Tibettan terrier who sat by me, literally, as I wrote, always ready to enjoy vicariously as I sampled the coffee, chocolate and wine that is not a part of her diet, settling for the occasional piece of bacon instead.

A Special Request From the Author

· ·

Having written this book in good faith, knowing full well my limitations, I will be very glad to receive your comments, corrections, experiences and notions. I promise to revise where needed, retract if I must and ask for forgiveness if all else fails. You may contact me at Mary@RoseCottagePress.com.

References

Coffee

Albin, A. (2/19/2009). **Coffee may protect against stroke**. Message posted to http://newsroom.ucla.edu/portal/ucla/coffee-may-protect-against-stroke-81879.aspx

Altman, M. (12/10/2010). Coffee causes strokes...sort of. Message posted to http://www.thecrimson.com/article/2010/12/15/coffee-stroke-risk-harvard/

Berkeley Wellness. (4/16/2013, **Decaf: A healthy choice?**

by berkeley Wellness | April 16, 2013. *Berkeley WEllness Newsletter,*

Berkowitz, S. (2011). **Coffee consumption and depression riskcomment on "Coffee, caffeine, and risk of depression among women"** . *Arch Intern Med., 171*(17), 1578-http://archinte.jamanetwork.com/article.aspx?articleid=1106300.

Bourgeois, K. (2013, 1/23/2013). In defence of coffee. Message posted to http://drkaleybourgeois.com/2013/01/23/in-defense-of-coffee/

Brice, M. (8/16/2012). **Seven surprising health benefits of coffee** . Message posted to http://www.medicaldaily.com/seven-surprising-health-benefits-coffee-241981#G5zpoqIgeJA7LrH2.99

*Bullet proof upgraded coffee.*http://www.bulletproofexec.com/coffee/

Caffeine and athletic performance. (2012,). Message posted to http://www.athletepharmacist.com/previousarticles/caffeine-and-athletic-performance

Church, R. (March/April 2011, Decaffeination process explained. *Roast, ,* 33.

*Coffee and health.*http://www.britishcoffeeassociation.org/

coffee_and_health/

Collazo-Clavell, M. (). **Does caffeine affect blood sugar?**. Message posted to http://www.mayoclinic.com/health/blood-sugar/AN01804

Davids, K. (1/2012). Low acid coffees. Message posted to http://www.coffeereview.com/article.cfm?ID=192

Eskenazi, B., Stapleton, A., Kharrazi, M., & Chee, W. (May 1999). Associations between maternal decaffeinated and caffeinated and fetal growth and gestational duration. *Epidemiology, 10*(3)

Gardner, A. (Health.com, 11/22/2011). Coffee may reduce women's cancer risk. Message posted to http://www.cnn.com/2011/11/22/health/coffee-reduces-cancer-risk

Hammond, A. (Australian Institute of Sport Fact Sheet, March 1, 2007.,). Careful with caffeine: The impact of caffeine on athletic performance.

careful with the caffeine: The impact of caffeine on athletic performance - see more at: Http://www.sportsmd.com/SportsMD_Articles/id/211.aspx#sthash.7xJaSikj.dpuf careful with the caffeine: The impact of caffeine on athletic performance - see more at: Http://www.sportsmd.com/SportsMD_Articles/id/211.aspx#sthash.7xJaSikj.dpuf. Message posted to http://www.sportsmd.com/SportsMD_Articles/id/211.aspx#sthash.7xJaSikj.dpbs

Harvard Health Letter. (2012,). **What is it about coffee?**. Message posted to http://www.health.harvard.edu/newsletters/Harvard_Health_Letter/2012/January/what-is-it-about-coffee

Health News Florida. (3/18/2013). **Daily green tea or coffee cuts stroke risk**. Message posted to health.wusf.usf.edu/post/daily-green-tea-or-coffee-cuts-stroke-risk

Healthfinder.gov. (2013,). **Can green tea, coffee reduce stroke risk?**. Message posted to http://www.healthfinder.gov/News/Article.

aspx?id=674435

Huffington Post Healthy Living. (12/18/2012). Coffee drinking linked with lower oral cancer death risk. Message posted to http:// www.huffingtonpost.com/2012/12/18/coffee-oral-cancer-throat-death_n_2317525.html

Huffington Post. (1/8/2013). **Soda consumption linked with higher depression risk in study (and the opposite goes for coffee)**. Message posted to http://www.huffingtonpost.com/2013/01/08/soda-depression-coffee-sweetened-beverages-drinks_n_2427150.html

Is decaffeinated coffee safe to drink?. (9/4/2012,). Message posted to http://goaskalice.columbia.edu/decaffeinated-coffee-safe-drink

Jang, Y., Kim, J., Shim, J., Kim, C., Jang, J., Lee, K., et al. (5/15/2013). Decaffeinated coffee prevents scopolamine-induced memory impairment in rats. *Behavioral Brain Research, 245*, 113-119.

Jaslow, R. (6/5/2012). Three cups of coffee per day might prevent alzheimer's in older adults. Message posted to http://www.cbsnews.com/8301-504763_162-57447490-10391704/three-cups-of-coffee-per-day-might-prevent-alzheimers-in-older-adults/

Kawalec, J. *The latest coffee research – does it stand up to scrutiny?*

Knowlton, S. (Health Guidance). Benefits of decaf coffee. Message posted to http://www.healthguidance.org/entry/15841/1/Benefits-of-Decaf-Coffee.html

Larsson, S., Virtamo, J., & Wolk, A. (2011). Coffee consumption and risk of stroke in women. *Stroke, 42*, 908-912-http://lib-sh.lsuhsc.edu/portals/factts/handouts/7_CoffeeConsumptionAndTheRiskOfStrokeInWomen.pdf.

Leibenluft, E., Fiero, P., Bartko, J., Moul, D., & Rosenthal, N. (Feb 1993). **Depressive symptoms and the self-reported use of** alcohol, caffeine, and carbohydrates in normal volunteers and four groups of psychiatric outpatients.. *Am J Psychiatry.*, *150*(2), 294-301.

Macintosh, Z. (5/25/2010).

Caffeine may counteract cognitive decline Message posted to http://www.livescience.com/6520-caffeine-counteract-cognitive-decline.html

McDaniel, L., McIntire, K., Streitz, C., Jackson, A., & Gaudet, L. (2009,). **The effects of caffeine on performance in sports: critical issues related to the effects of caffeine on athlete's performance**. Message posted to http://www.brianmac.co.uk/articles/article058.htm

McMillen, M. (9/26/2011). **For women, risk of depression falls as coffee intake rises**. Message posted to www.cnn.com/2011/09/26/health/women-depression-coffee/index.html

Mostofsky, E., Rice, M., Levitan, E., & Mittleman, M. (2012). Habitual coffee consumption and risk of heart failure: A dose-response meta-analysis. *Circulation Heart Failure,*

Mostofsky, E., Schlaug, G., Mukamal, K., Rosamond, W., & Mittleman, M. (2010). **Coffee and acute ischemic stroke onset: The stroke onset study.**. *Neurology.*, *75*(18), 1583-8.

Mount Sinai Medical Center. (2/1/2012, **Decaffeinated coffee may help improve memory function and reduce risk of diabetes**. *Science Daily,*

Ohnaka, K., Ikeda, M., Maki, T., Okada, T., Shimazoe, T., Adachi, M., et al. (2012). **Effects of 16-week consumption of caffeinated and decaffeinated instant coffee on glucose metabolism in a randomized controlled trial**. *J Nutr Metab. 2012; 2012: 207426.,*

Parnell, J. (2012, 3/122012). **Wake up and smell the coffee coffee consumptiuon and risk of chronic diseases: Changing our views**. Message posted to http://no-baloney.com/2012/03/12/

wake-up-and-smell-the-coffee/

Pham, N., Nanri, A., Kurotani, K., Kuwahara, K., Kume, A., Sato, M., et al. (March 2013). Green tea and coffee consumption is inversely associated with depressive symptoms in a japanese working population. *Public Health Nutrition, 4,* 1-9.

Rafetto, M., Cherniske, S., & French, G. (2005). *Effect of decaffeinated coffee on health.*

Research on coffee and cancer website. http://www.coffeeand-health.org/research-centre/cancer/

ROSENGREN, A., & WILHELMSEN, L. (1991). Coffee, coronary heart disease and mortality in middle-aged swedish men: Findings from the primary prevention study. *Journal of Internal Medicine, 230*(1), 67-71.

Ruusunen, A., Lehto, S., Tolmunen, T., Mursu, J., Kaplan, G., & Voutilainen, S. (August 2013). Coffee, tea and caffeine intake and the risk of severe depression in middle-aged finnish men: The kuopio ischaemic heart disease risk factor study. *Public Health Nutrition, 13*(8), 1215-1220.

Salzberg, S. (12/23/2012). Have another cup of coffee-it's good for you. Message posted to http://www.forbes.com/sites/stevensalzberg/2012/12/23/have-another-cup-of-coffee-its-good-for-you/

Science News. (6/28/2011). **Mystery ingredient in coffee boosts protection against alzheimer's disease, study finds**. Message posted to http://www.sciencedaily.com/releases/2011/06/110621093301.htm

Tavani, A., & La Vecchia, C. (October 2004,). Coffee, decaffeinated coffee, tea and cancer of the colon and rectum: A review of epidemiological studies, 1990-2003 *Cancer Causes and Control, 15*(8), 743-757.

Trunk, D. **UF experts: Decaffeinated coffee is not caffeine-free.** *10/10/2006,* van Dusseldorp, M., Smits, P., Thien, T., & Katan, M. (1989). **Effect of decaffeinated versus regular coffee on blood pressure. A 12-week, double-blind trial.**. *Hypertension., 14,* 563-569.

von Dam, R., Willett, W., Manson, J., & Hu, F. (Feb. 2006). Caffeinated and caffeine-free beverages and risk of type 2 diabetes. *Diabetes Care, 29*(2), 398-403.

Wedick, N., Mantzoros, C., Ding, E., Brennan, A., Rosner, B., Rimm, E., et al. **The effects of caffeinated and decaffeinated coffee on sex hormone-binding globulin and endogenous sex hormone levels: A randomized controlled trial.**

Wenk, G. (5/23/2011, Why decaf coffee is just as healthy. *Psychology Today,*

Wheeler, C. (April 1998,). Caffeine: Is it friend or foe of martial artists? Message posted to http://books.google.com/books?id=0tkDAAAAMBAJ&pg=PA26&dq=effects+of+coffee+on+strength+and+endurance-all+around+athletic+ability&hl=en&sa=X&ei=w2BEUa_dJNK14AP6uYHABg&ved=0CDsQ6AEwAQ#v=onepage&q=effects%20of%20coffee%20on%20strength%20and%20endurance-all%20around%20athletic%20ability&f=false

Wheeler, M. (1/12/2011). **Why coffee protects against diabetes researchers discover molecular mechanism behind drink's prophylactic effect.** Message posted to http://newsroom.ucla.edu/portal/ucla/why-coffee-protects-against-diabetes-190743.aspx

Wood, S. (11/17/2005,). **Decaf coffee raises LDL cholesterol** Message posted to http://www.medscape.com/viewarticle/788017?t=1&topol=1

Chocolate

Aubry, A. (3/26/2012,). Does A chocolate habit help keep you lean? Message posted to http://www.npr.org/blogs/thesalt/2012/03/26/149407484/does-a-chocolate-habit-help-keep-you-lean

Freeman, S. Is chocolate an aphrodisiac? Message posted to http://science.howstuffworks.com/innovation/edible-innovations/chocolate-aphrodisiac.htm

Goran, M., Ulijaszek, S., & Ventura, E. (2013). High fructose corn syrup and diabetes prevalence: A global perspective. *Global Public Health, 8*(1), 55-64.

Gutierrez, D. (6/21/2013, **Reduce your cholesterol with chocolate: Research**. *Natural News.Com,*

Hub Pages. **How to sleep better - chocolate helps you sleep.** Message posted to http://hubpages.com/hub/How-To-Sleep-Better

Mail Online. Why hot chocolate is perfect at bedtime. Message posted to http://www.dailymail.co.uk/femail/article-4982/Why-hot-chocolate-perfect-bedtime.html

MindPower Blog. (3/22/2010,). **Hot chocolate: Bed time drink or disturbed sleep?**. Message posted to http://mind-power-book.com/blog/Hot-Chocolate-Bed-Time-Drink-or-Disturbed-Sleep

Mitchell, E., Slettenaar, M., vd Meer, N., Transler, C., Jans, L., Quadt, F., et al. (10/24/2011). Differential contributions of theobromine and caffeine on mood, psychomotor performance and blood pressure. *Physiol Behav., 104*(5), 816-822.

Mostofsky E, Levitan EB, Wolk A, Mittleman MA. (9/3/2010). Chocolate intake and incidence of heart failure: A population-based prospective study of middle-aged and elderly women. . *Circulation Heart Failure, 3*(5), 612-616.

Reynolds, G. (8/3/2011,). How chocolate can help your workout . Message posted to http://well.blogs.nytimes.com/2011/08/03/how-chocolate-can-help-your-workout/?_r=1

Robbins, K. (8/9/2011,). **Eating dark chocolate could improve physical endurance**. Message posted to http://www.delish.com/food/recalls-reviews/dark-chocolate-improves-physical-endurance-study-ucsd

Yalung, B. (1/12/2009,). **Chocolate can be a sleep disruptor**. Message posted to sleepzine.com/sleep-news/chocolate-can-be-a-sleep-disruptor/

Wine

Godman, H. (9/12/2012,). **Non-alcoholic red wine may lower blood pressure**. Message posted to http://www.health.harvard.edu/blog/non-alcoholic-red-wine-may-lower-blood-pressure-201209125296

Griva, V. (11/28/2007,). **Red wine protects against food-borne germs**
. Message posted to http://jamaica-gleaner.com/gleaner/20071128/health/health6.html

Grogan, M. (). **Does grape juice offer the same heart benefits as red wine?**. Message posted to http://www.mayoclinic.com/health/food-and-nutrition/AN00576

Mann, D. (9/6/2012,). **Non-alcoholic red wine may boost heart health**. Message posted to http://www.webmd.com/hypertension-high-blood-pressure/news/20120906/nonalcoholic-red-wine-may-boost-heart-health

Naik, G. (8/30/2012,). **Big calorie cuts don't equal longer life, study suggests**. Message posted to http://online.wsj.com/article/SB10000872396390444772804577619394017185860.html

Neporent, L. (9/7/2012,). **Drink to your heart's content -- if it's nonalcoholic**. Message posted to http://abcnews.go.com/Health/Diet/red-wine-minus-alcohol-lower-blood-pressure-study/story?id=17173121

Nutrition in exercise and sport, 3rd edition.

R. Corder, R., Mullen, W., Khan, N., Marks, S., Wood, E., Carrier, M., et al. (11/30/2006). **Oenology: Red wine procyanidins and vascular health**. *Nature, 444*, 566.

Roberts, M. (7/8/2012,). **Drinking alcohol, even in moderation, 'a dementia risk'**. Message posted to http://www.bbc.co.uk/news/health-18856658

Three glasses of champagne a week keeps dementia away! india.com Health May 6, 2013. (India.com Health, 5/6/2013). Message posted to http://health.india.com/news/three-glasses-of-champagne-a-week-keeps-dementia-away/

Wagner, H. (12/8/2004,). **Red wine limits effect of cardiac fibrosis**. Message posted to http://www.medicalnewstoday.com/releases/17456.php

CPSIA information can be obtained
at www.ICGtesting.com
Printed in the USA
FFOW04n0738231013

2114FF